40D
as a
Cit
Caveman

In order to take two steps forward in health and fitness,
one must take a step back in time…
the City Caveman way.

Michael Jarosky
and Annie Clark

For legal purposes, I have to list those who made contributions in order to get this book printed. But, I must further state a genuine thank you, as those listed below did more than just their jobs…they were a cool, honest and fun group to work with. Anybody going down the self-publishing road should also seek out their friendly and helpful services.

…………….

This second edition published in Australia, 2008.

Photography

Before photos – Avi Ohana at Celebrity Vogue Photography, Sydney
After photos – Mofid Guirguis at Freeman Studio, Sydney
Workout photos – Trevor Martin at Trevor Martin Photography, Sydney
Workout model – Kali Holmes, Sydney
Photo editing – Jessica Kalieta, New Jersey (USA)

Design

Cover design – Chai Lim at chinc.dzine, Sydney
Page layout design – J&M Typesetting

Nutrition Advisor

Rita Cozzi at Rita Erba-Cozzi and Associates, Sydney

Editing and Proofreading

Editing – Analee Matthews at All Smiles Creative, Sydney
Proofreading – Tim Clark at Ripe Off The Press, Melbourne
Project management – Libby Rule at Ripe Off The Press, Melbourne

Printing and Distribution

Printed and bound in Australia by Trojan Press
Distributed by Dennis Jones & Associates

To our families

Contents

Foreword

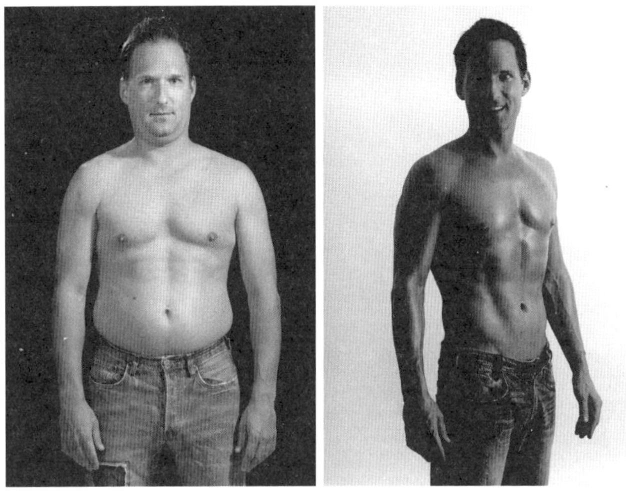

A book's foreword is typically written by someone other than the author. However, I, Mike Jarosky, am writing this foreword because in forty days I *have* become a new person, with a new body, newfound health, and a new life.

I am truly different, and I love it.

I never blamed the marketers at McDonald's for my love handles, and I was never going to sue Pizza Hut because of my man boobs. I was unhealthy because I chose an indulgent lifestyle that needed to stop, *immediately*.

I was on the cusp of turning 35 years old, and I needed to make a serious change in my lifestyle, so I took on the challenge of living like a caveman (I'll explain later what I mean by that) for just forty days, and it changed my life and my body entirely.

The same plan can work for you.

This book tells the story of my 40-day journey, including my daily progress and my feelings along the way. But, at the core of this tale are also workouts, recipes and a health plan that any man or woman of any age can undertake, and that *will* work.

I did not achieve my successful transformation alone. Like many memorable journeys, this one was undertaken with a mate. For me, Annie Clark was that friend. Annie is a Sydney-based fitness professional and trained psychologist who worked out with me and supported me through the tougher parts of the 40-day program. And so together, we created the City Caveman Plan.

We hope this book, and my journey, will inspire and motivate you to become your own City Caveman, and to achieve life-changing health in just forty days.

Like I did.

Have fun, and best of luck!

Mike Jarosky
City Caveman

The City Caveman Plan

The City Caveman Plan can be summarised easily: healthy and fresh eating with effective, straightforward workouts.

Now, don't think I am a nutbag, as I never planned on hunting and gathering my own food, carving meat and cracking field nuts. Simply put, the City Caveman Plan is based around the concepts of 'simple' and 'fresh', both in the kitchen and at the gym.

Cavemen ate fresh foods, not the fried, processed junk food that is full of who-knows-what chemicals, like our foods are today. And this is the very crux of the City Caveman Plan.

As for workouts, the same applies; simple, simple, simple one-hour workouts that target the whole body. The workout plans were developed so they are suitable for young or old, males or females; they are not complex, yet are extremely effective.

So there you have it. The secret to the entire program is now yours. Now, should you put the book down and get started? Absolutely not! Because while the answer is pretty simple, the process of executing the plan and achieving real change is not, and that is what this book is about. After all, you may be able to buck the trend of futuristic fat loss plans, but the ability to buck the trend of your own abusive, unhealthy lifestyle is where the real challenge lies.

If you are reading this book because you are feeling tired of your body, tired of your over-consumption and tired of feeling like shit about yourself, then you are on the right track. Because that is exactly how I felt when I decided to create the City Caveman Plan. So if that's how you *are* feeling, then the time is probably right for you to give up the excuses and commit to making a change. I successfully put down the beers and bypassed the kebab shops, and I took my love handles and man-boobs into that intimidating space called a gym. And I survived! As a result, my body and my life changed remarkably. But the best part? I gave myself another chance at having a life I can actually enjoy.

As you read this book, you will probably identify with the challenges that I went through, some of which were physical, and a lot of which were emotional. The bottom line is, though: if I can do it, so can you.

How to Prepare for the City Caveman Plan

During my forty days as a City Caveman, I learned so many things, many of which could have eased some of the tough spots in the early days. So, in this section I want to share some of these 'golden nuggets'.

1 Game Day

Before my Caveman days, my workouts consisted mainly of going for a run, dragging a heavyweight hangover all the way. Therefore, when the City Caveman Plan came along, in order to successfully make it through my training sessions, I knew I had to mentally prepare myself, because there was no personal trainer waiting to motivate me for all forty days; I was accountable to only myself on a daily basis. So, to enter the gym as a chubby chap, I developed an 'It's Game Day' approach, similar to when athletes take to the playing field for competition. Silly? Maybe so, but for me it worked. It was kind of like this switch went off in my head, which enabled me to focus myself for just one hour each day, so I could make it through the workout.

I do believe we all have this zone; it's that place in our minds where we feel motivated to achieve our goals. Maybe it's the constant reminder of how embarrassing your (soon-to-be) before-photo looks, or the news from your doctor that you should prepare yourself for a future of serious health issues. Whatever your reason for taking the City Caveman Plan on, you store that reason in that zone, so when your motivation wilts, you can tap into it and power through your training.

2 Battles

During the forty days, your favourite soft drink is off limits, forget about kebabs, and you'll have to miss the Saturday night piss-ups at the local pub. Make no mistake, you *will* be battling.

In making a lifestyle change, it is not just the new things that you will integrate into your life (training regularly and eating healthy), it is also about the things you might be accustomed to giving in to, which you will now have to give up. And this is a *battle*. I found it difficult giving up those cheeky niceties on a daily basis, so I had to learn how to substitute the physical pleasure with the mental reward of knowing that every time I said 'no' to a Coke, or didn't have a beer, or didn't indulge in a row of Tim Tams, that I was winning the battles one-by-one, and improving my health day-by-day, *battle-by-battle*.

These battles are everywhere, and over forty days you will face some of the challenges that I did, and some of your very own. It is your task to win them all and, in doing so, you will be successfully fast-tracking your health to optimal condition.

3 10 Days at a Time

You might be thinking, 'Forty days is a long time. Can I really do this?' Well, let me help you discard that thinking by introducing a different line of thinking.

Instead of thinking about *forty days*, change your thinking to focus on ten-day increments. Can you do this for ten days? Of course you can. So once you finish the initial ten-day period, you will already be feeling better, both mentally and physically, so committing to one more period of ten days will be easier than the first. And so, too, will the next ten days, and the next. You may not see it yet, but once you start feeling the difference and seeing results, the momentum will kick in naturally, and your motivation will come easily.

Of course, during these ten-day blocks, you will still have your battles and challenges, and you will come face-to-face with your demons. But you will find your groove when you and your body start changing for the better.

If you start to wane or feel overwhelmed by the duration of the City Caveman Plan, remind yourself that forty days of healthy living, as compared to – in my instance – thirty-five years of poor living, is a tiny percentage of a life that will be extended after you complete the Plan. Take it head on, just ten days at a time, and you will successfully reach Day 40 of the City Caveman Plan.

4 Excitement and Doubt

I hope I am correct in guessing you have a mixture of emotions at this point of the program. You're feeling excited to start your Plan, but doubt or fear may linger in the wings. That *excitement* is fantastic. Riding this nervous energy will definitely help you in the first week and even into the second. Throughout the forty days there will definitely be ups and downs, pleasure and frustration, but feeling excited to commence means you know that you are onto a good thing, and that a new and healthy life is within your grasp.

Your dual feeling of being doubtful and nervous is completely normal. When you decide to embark on an unfamiliar journey, it is natural to feel unsettled, but take heart in knowing that, once you start the program and begin to achieve results, those doubts will soon disappear.

5 This is Not a Diet

If you want to go on a diet, please pass this book on to someone else. If you own a television, you already know that diets don't work, and I am not the type to sell you the next great diet with promises of short-term miracle fat loss!

Instead, the City Caveman Plan is exactly that – a plan. It is a method to change your lifestyle to assist in changing your health. It is not a book about what you can or can't eat but, rather, it is an educational tool to help you understand that by eating fresh, tasty food and undertaking regular, simple workouts, your body and mind will thank you in ways that you will love. The City Caveman Plan is not about deprivation. I grew up with a dad who owned a restaurant in Chicago, so food has always been part of my life, and when I need steak, well, I need steak! I also enjoy bread, so I've ensured that the Plan includes bread. The City Caveman Plan is one that food-lovers can take on, while still loving their food!

That said, by taking on the City Caveman Plan, you will alter the way you view food. If you are what I call a *pleasure eater*, like I am, then every meal has to be packed with flavour, consumed in huge portions, and that usually equates to food packed with sodium, salt, fat and unknown chemicals that will all pile on the kilos. The City Caveman Plan will transfer you from a pleasure eater to a fresh, healthy energy eater.

I will admit, this transfer was one of the harder battles I faced during my forty days because I looooove the flavour in food. Before I embarked on the City Caveman Plan, a meal of chicken parmigiana, garlic bread, fried calamari, too much wine, a big slice of tiramisu and some cheese would have been the norm for me. I never wanted the flavours to stop, so I didn't stop eating. But, during the City Caveman Plan, I realised that meals full of fat, grease, sugar and sodium were contributing to my sluggish behaviour, lack of desire to be active, bad skin and certainly my bulging gut. It really was time to stop.

The City Caveman Plan is geared toward transforming that pleasure consumption into a love for healthy food that your body, your skin and your mind will enjoy and reap benefits from; it's about consuming food that will give you energy throughout the day and energy where you need it most – during your workouts.

6 The Goal

Forget about obtaining Brad Pitt's or Angelina Jolie's body in a month's time, because if Hollywood hasn't called yet, they probably won't, right?

Think more about attaining what I call the 'Happy-Healthy Zone'. It's that place in our mind that makes us happy and confident with our bodies and who we are. It's not about perfection or having a body that should be on a magazine cover. Throw that thought right out the window because perfection is realistically unobtainable. Instead, rethink your goals and strive to be in that zone where *you* feel comfortable with *your* body, *your* mind and *your* overall health. For me, it was all about having the confidence to look good in jeans and a t-shirt, and feeling comfortable in a swimsuit at the beach.

By keeping my goal simple and realistic, I actually managed to exceed my own expectations by the end of forty days. I found my Happy-Healthy Zone with the City Caveman Plan, and it's the happiest place I've ever been!

ze

As you take on the City Caveman Plan, I guarantee at one point or another, you will see the following take place in a gym:

> *There will be a muscle-clad person in the gym using 50kgs to perform an arm curl. Yet, instead of only using the bicep muscles and arms, the back, legs and chest are all recruited in order for that weight to be lifted up and down.*

Why do people in the gym take on too much weight for the exercise they're doing? Because they think it makes them look impressive. However, if that same person decreased that weight by half and used controlled, precise arm movements that only challenged the bicep muscles to move that weight up and down, then not only would the risk of injury be significantly reduced, but a better workout would be had. And the results from that exercise would be achieved faster. Don't let ego control your workout, or your results may take longer to obtain.

I learned, during my City Caveman Plan, that it is not weight, strength, show-manship or ego that gets the best workout, but instead, it is all about the 'squeeze.'

When I am in the gym, next to that musclehead, I will happily take my 10kg weights and use them with correct form and the right motion, by *squeezing* my muscles in order to make that weight move throughout its range of motion. Continuing on, I *squeeze* out my ab muscles during sit-ups, and I *squeeze* out my leg muscles during leg extensions. The squeeze allows me to increase the intensity of my workouts, without taking on more weight or having to stay in the gym for more hours.

Your new mantra? Squeezing works.

8 Is it Easy?

Leaning to the left, picking up the phone and ordering a large meatlover's pizza, then consuming it; that is easy. Living a life with chronic heart problems or diabetes – that is hard.

Deep down, we all want achieving health and transforming our lives to be easy! But, if you search deep down into your soul, you know that turning your life around has to be a challenging process if it's going to be a permanent change. The ability to make that change in one's life and move from unfit and unhealthy to a fit and healthy stage is not easy; it's more what I consider a fun, exciting *challenge*.

Unfortunately, there are no cutting corners, there are no shortcuts – it is just about healthy eating and efficient workouts and the challenges that lie within adopting these things into your everyday life. Trust me, there were times during the City Caveman Plan where I could have physically strangled a guy on the street holding a gooey cheese-filled lamb kebab for just one bite!

There were also some days where my legs just felt 'off,' so going for a run was the last thing I wanted to do. It will not be easy, but just remember that those ups and downs are an unavoidable part of the process. The solution to achieving your goal is to continue to focus on what you are trying to achieve; leaving a lifestyle that doesn't serve you well, and creating a new healthy life for yourself. When you feel overwhelmed or unmotivated, remember this.

On the flip side, because the process is so challenging, the rewards will be HUGE! For me, some (but not all) of the benefits I received during and after my City Caveman Plan were:

- clear skin
- fresh and bright looking eyes
- healthy times on the toilet
- improved performances in my running times and overall fitness
- a healthier and more toned-looking body
- looking younger
- nothing jiggling or wobbling on my body anymore
- much better sex
- being 'fit tired' at night rather than 'fat/bloated tired'
- no more week-long hangovers
- no more sugar highs and lows

- improved strength
- improved cardiovascular fitness
- improved mind/body confidence

These rewards are just some of the pleasures you'll receive after forty days of battling. Remember, all hardships can be overshadowed by awesome results, and my new body, my new wardrobe, my new smile and my new life are all fine examples of the reward far outweighing the effort required to reach the end goal.

9 Sacrifice and Time

So at this point, you might be thinking, 'How can I fit anything else into my current schedule?'

By taking on the City Caveman Plan, you have a desire to shift your lifestyle into the *Change Phase* (I'll talk more about this shortly). To do so, you must be willing to make some sacrifices. So the bottom line is, *you need to make the time to take on the Plan and what it entails*.

In order for you to sacrifice the eating/drinks nights out, plan your eating for the week and undertake the workouts, you will need to learn how to ignore *beer and peer* pressure and start thinking about your *blood* pressure.

During the City Caveman Plan, I guarantee that you will sleep better and have more energy and that at some stage you will start *wanting* to work out. Statistics can be annoying, but a one-hour workout, six times a week, takes up only about four per cent of our entire week. We can all make time for important things when we need to!

Remind yourself: each day of the Plan is about your body, your health and your life.

10 Accountability

We will look at the accountability of your health in three stages, but be warned: I won't pull any punches because there is only one person who got you into your current state, and there is only one person who can get you out of it – you.

a *Pre-City Caveman Plan*

You are currently not in the body or the health that *you* want because of the choices *you* have made about *your* food intake and *your* lack of exercise.

b *City Caveman Plan*

By taking on the City Caveman Plan, *you* are the only person who can make a long-lasting health and lifestyle change in *your* life.

c *Post-City Caveman Plan*

When the City Caveman Plan is complete *you* will have the tools and knowledge necessary to control *your* lifestyle and maintain *your* life, the healthy way.

My point on accountability is that this is *your* life, *your* health and *your* wellbeing. As I mentioned earlier, neither McDonald's nor any other third party could be my excuse as to why I was unfit and unhealthy. The reason for my poor health, and the only reason, was me.

This is why supplement pills and other fat loss gizmos don't work, because instead of truly understanding what we are putting into our bodies, we take the lazy approach and shift accountability to the pill by thinking, 'Well, maybe this pill can take the weight off for me.' Wrong!

During the City Caveman Plan, it is critical that you learn how to take accountability for your eating and your workouts. To help you become accountable, part of the City Caveman Plan recommends you use an accountability mechanism that will keep you on track on a daily basis. This mechanism will be attached to your mirror, as it was mine, and it will allow you to hold yourself accountable for each of your forty days.

As I've said, there is no hand-holding through the forty days and there are no wondrous potions that can do the hard yards for you. It is up to you to follow t he plan and look yourself in the mirror each day with the satisfaction of being able to say 'Today I battled, and I won.' Hold yourself fully accountable, and you cannot fail.

11 Post-forty days

The end of Day 40 will not actually be a finish line as such. Instead, it will be the start of a new, controlled beginning. Think about it. When you're done with your forty days, you will have created newfound health, a better body and a new life, so it really is just the beginning.

And finally…

12 Enjoy!

I know it all sounds like a lot of hard work, and I won't lie: sometimes it is. But don't forget to enjoy, enjoy, enjoy this journey as well. Positive change is something to appreciate and celebrate, and becoming fit and healthy opens up a whole new world.

I now enjoy and appreciate active Saturdays in the sun by the ocean, long hikes and the potential for active holidays, rather than weekends and vacations based solely around food and alcohol intake. The City Caveman Plan showed me a new way to live and, believe me, it is a far more enjoyable lifestyle.

When I look back now, I did enjoy the challenge. I enjoyed the ups and the downs, and I really enjoy my new body. I love having a clear mind, and I really enjoy buying and wearing my new clothes! My fitness has given me a new life, and my new life has the possibility of taking me in any direction I want. It's hard to believe that at 35 years of age, I feel like I have discovered a new type of freedom and have only just started living.

So, there you have it. Those are the tips that can help your journey through the City Caveman Plan.

By turning the page, you are confirming that you *do* want to change your life and your health for the better, and that you *are* fully committed to the process, for at least forty days.

This book has been designed to help you as you progress through the 40-day Plan. So, during your preparation stages, read up to Day Zero, and then as each day in your journey arrives, read what I experienced on that day when I did the program. We are all individuals, so, chances are, your experiences and feelings will differ from mine; however, I am sure you will encounter many similar battles, so my daily diary should help provide some support and serve as a reminder that you are not alone and what you are experiencing is not unusual.

Therefore I hope my daily diary will aid your forty days and you identify Annie as your fitness guide and me as your workout buddy, folly friend and kitchen helper.

Have fun and best of luck!

1

Introduction

Next month, on June 23rd, I will be 35 years old.

I just arrived home from a workout. Well, not a workout by a personal trainer's standard. I went to the gym with the intention of running five kilometres, doing some abdominal work, and maybe throwing a few weights around here and there. Add to that a steam, shower and a nice shave, and I figured I would start my day feeling fresh as a daisy. Unfortunately, it didn't quite happen that way.

Today is Saturday, and I woke up with a striking hangover. Last night, I arrived home in my bed around 3am after more than a few wines, four beers and a couple of rum and colas. It was a mate's birthday party; there was good food, fun chatting, flirting and a bit of dancing in one of those swanky bars in the seedy-yet-trendy part of Sydney. Post-drinks I ran into my favourite fast food joint, downed a value meal number whatever, and to pour a little more petrol on the fire, I found a 7-Eleven with one last beef 'Traveller's Pie,' of which I ended up spilling a quarter down my shirt.

I woke at 10am today with that hideously ill feeling. I fumbled to put my workout clothes on and filled my gym bag with my post-shower gear. I popped two tablets I bought at the local vitamin shop that are supposed to increase my metabolism (I think they help me lose weight). And since I was feeling extra fragile, for good measure I stopped at the local convenience store to down a Red Bull, hoping that my modern medical science concoction of metabolism pills and energy drink would give me the right buzz to hit the treadmill with full force.

Boy. Was I wrong.

By the time I arrived at the gym, I felt like a living, walking zombie. A stop in the gym toilet was a necessity as last night's meal(s) demanded to see the light of day. After this, I was ready to begin my workout, which started with my mandatory three minute look-around stretch/perve. And then I was ready to go.

Or so I thought.

Instead of five kilometres, I ran 2.3 kilometres at half my normal speed as the pounding on the treadmill was doing my head in, and there were no good music videos on to keep me entertained. Then, instead of my ab workout, I hit the water cooler; and, finally, instead of throwing a few weights around, I pranced right past the bench press and into the locker room to gather my gear and head out for a stack of pancakes with two eggs and an orange juice. And then, off home I went.

And that was the conclusion of my Saturday workout. No sweating, no exhaustion, no…nothing, really.

Okay, let me back right up because I must sound like quite a lazy pig. But the truth is, growing up in Chicago, my brother and I were the healthiest kids on the block, undertaking sports all day and healthy eating at mealtimes thanks to a great mum.

But, like most kids during childhood, a healthy lunch was never really on my mind. Rectangular gooey pizza, that yummy turkey on white bread oozing with mashed potatoes and gravy, and French fries covered in nacho cheese – it all sounded so exciting. The lunches my mum prepared and sent us off to school with were about as fun as a tooth extraction: brown bread with turkey and tomato, dried fruit with nuts, skim milk in that smelly cardboard container, and a banana with numerous shades of bruise from the beating it took on its way to school. *None* of the other children wanted to trade lunches with me.

Those years were healthy, full of sports, and rarely did a sick day come. I never put on a kilogram of weight unless it was due to playing baseball or basketball – quite the American fairytale.

But then came university and the opportunity to be on my own for the first time. Living outside the confines of the Jarosky household, I was free to eat whatever I pleased. As long as I obtained good grades, I allowed myself all the underage alcohol I could consume, and I had an absolute blast shopping at the local grocery store for sugary cookies, ice cream, fried chicken dinners and icing-coated apple-filled pastries. It was all so yummy! I was 21, I was away at University, I was having girls over, and I had a fridge full of cold beer and tasty goodies. Life seemed fantastic.

That was, until one day during a trip home when mum said, ‘Michael, your butt is getting bigger.’

It all happens to us at some age. Eventually, our young person’s fast metabolism abandons us, and the lack of working out and avoiding sports mixed with questionable eating results in weight gain.

In the years that followed, my weight fluctuated like a yo-yo. I’d gain a few kilograms here, work out and lose a few there. My business degree led to a great job in financial consulting, and our ‘boys club’ of workmates was always out and about eating, drinking and overdoing it. From enormous steaks in Chicago, to vodka martinis and crème bruleé in New York City, we ate and drank it all.

During a rare day off in New York City, my boss, Tim, and I played a game of racquetball. It lasted about four minutes because after that long, Tim was panting like a fish out of water and I was in hysterics. We left that racquetball court after calling it a day and me leading at 3 to 2 – points, not games! At this point in time I was so chunky I couldn’t even button the shorts I’d purchased just three months earlier. My passport photo was taken that same year. What a poor reminder of the beginning of my double chin. I was 25 years old but I looked 40. And I was reminded of this every time I travelled for the next ten years!

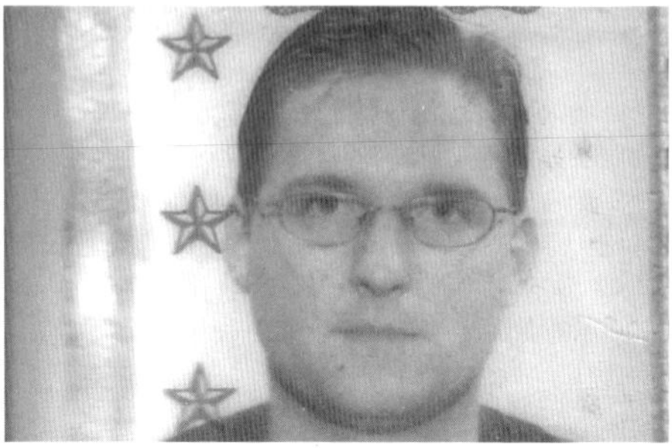

The weight continued to come and go. Over the subsequent years, I always held a gym membership, running or riding the bike with the only real goal being to negate my poor eating and the prior night's drinking. I certainly was not ultra fit, and I was not ultra fat – I was just 'comfortable.'

While working in the financial consulting field, I put my career and big weekends ahead of my health and my fitness. And when I did try to make a change, I always did it half-arsed. For example, around the time my passport photo was taken, I was on one of my workout *kicks*, and my brother saw me in a sweaty daze, jogging home carrying my backpack. He probably assumed I was carrying my gear back from the gym, so he honked, and said he'd drive me the rest of the way. Moments after I sat in the car, he sniffed, and asked, 'What's that smell?' To which, I replied, 'I've got a KFC six-piece extra crispy in my backpack.' Health and fitness was not really a priority for me.

Ten years on from this KFC moment, I live in amazing Australia, where the freshest of food is available, yet so too are my tasty, cheeky and fatty favourites. Drinking is like a national sport to many Australians and also one of my own favourites, so I fast developed a lifestyle where wine over dinner on Wednesday, led to Thursday night city drinks, which, in turn, resulted in Friday, Saturday and Sunday hangovers. And, of course, when somebody puts the call out for 'a few quiet ones' on a Sunday, Monday, or Tuesday, they could usually count on my presence!

I still go to the gym regularly, but there is no real goal other than to work off the damage that I do to my body at the bar and the snack shop. I go right past the spin class, have a look in the boxercise classes, and shyly walk past the Arnie wannabes in the weight room. I don my American baseball cap, my trusty iPod, and I zone out on a treadmill for my hamster-like running workout. I am truly goal-less and, if I'm really honest, my body shows it.

My Internet dating profile from the past always said I have an 'athletic' body type, but I know that I selected that option with 'oh, I played sports in high school, and therefore I have an athletic build' in mind. My meek workouts and big nights out have left me with quite a below-average body. I'm not *athletic*; in fact, I'm far closer to *pathetic*. The love handles are there, the man boobs are starting to take shape, and the sight of me, shirtless, wearing a pair of jeans is *not* pretty.

I am not huge, but I am far from fit. I am more like Jack Black; you know, where there is a solid portion of chub on my body, but I try to deny it's there and so only send photos home to Mom during my not-so-fat stage, or when the angle is just right to hide my second chin and obvious belly.

In order to still look presentable, I mastered the I-am-not-that-fat-hiding techniques, such as:

- **a** The *suck-in move*, where I never allow my full gut to bow outward by ensuring I always have a little suck-in of the gut and a little push-out of the chest.
- **b** The *untucked shirt move*, which ensures I never allow my belly to be exposed via a tucked-in shirt and muffin-top gut hanging over my belt.
- **c** The *high towel move*, where I wrap the post-shower towel above my belly button to hide my gut.
- **d** The *S.O.F.A (Shirt Over Fat Arse) move*, whereby I tie a jacket around my waist to cover up that extra waistline and saggy bum (a move, often more popular with females than males).
- **e** The *suit move*, which allows me to wear a suit so I can relax underneath numerous layers.
- **f** The *no-beach move,* which means never allowing myself to be seen on a beach, topless, or in a swimsuit.

Regardless of whatever disguise techniques I deploy during the day, at the end of that day, in the mirror, I am exposed. The mirror cannot lie to me, and I am not happy with what it says. It tells me that I am not well; it tells me that I am not comfortable with my body; and it tells me that now is the time to make a change.

> *The mirror is telling me that I am hung over, that I am ill, and that I need a nap. That mirror is telling me that I need to make some changes. That mirror is telling me that next month, on the 23rd of June, I will be 35 years old, and I feel like shit.*

2

Assessing My Current Situation

I am at a stage where I am through feeling the way I feel and looking the way I look. Today is the day I am going to do something about it. Yes, yes, yes, how many times have I said this before, right? Quite a few actually. From the 'Oh, I will start it on the first of *next* month' to the 'Just one more Sunday pizza night and then I will start with my fitness challenge,' I have made every excuse to deny and delay making the change my body craves.

But today, today, TODAY I am making a commitment to make that damn change!

I know that deep inside I have a fit man waiting to be released. Bah! That sounds like another cliché, doesn't it? All those clichés I have heard the fatties on Oprah talk about, and now I am one of them and I am saying the same, damn things. However, I am done *chasing* that fit person. The time is now that I *become* him. He is what I want to be, he is who I aspire to be, and he is my goal. I *will* bridge the gap to become him.

I do know what it takes to get fit. It takes a plan, and the committed execution of that plan. Add a heavy dose of common sense about eating and drinking, and the desire to change, and I can achieve my goal to be that fit man.

It really is that simple, isn't it?

I have swallowed the diet pills and done the eight-minute abs videos. (Okay, I probably only did two minutes in total, but I gave it a shot!) And I have been to the bookstore where there are shelves of books on health, diet and fitness. Yet all of these books are from some cheesy-smiling personal trainer, model, or a doctor. Ohhhhhhh, they can give their advice, healthy eating tips and turn-you-into-Arnold fitness advice, but do they really know how I feel inside? Do they really know what it's like to be a fatty and how hard it is to give up food? Do they really know how hard it is to truly become motivated to change?

I am neither a doctor, nor a model, nor a personal trainer. But I am real. And I am really going to try and make a change. I recall from movies and television shows that the first step in rehabilitating one's mind and body is admitting there's a problem. If that is the case, then I admit it: *I, Mike Jarosky, am a fatty.*

My daily behaviour has become too consistent: abbreviated exercise with no real workout plan, high-fat/low nutrition meals, followed by night-time drinks and a resulting hangover. And today was no different. My attempt at a five kilometre run ended after two kilometres before I hit the locker room for the Lazy Man's Triathlon (a poo, a steam room and a shower). I left the gym to go and meet a few friends for some Sunday beers at the local, and so I am writing this with the pleasant, cheeky effects of a six-schooner buzz.

I want to change. Yet I continue to do the same things that disallow this change. I eat poorly, I drink too much and my exercise regime is a joke.

The financial and strategic consultant I am trained to be tells me I need to make a plan to change because what I am doing now is not serving me well. I realise that the first thing to do is examine my current lifestyle and see where changes need to be made, although I already know that I need to start with my eating and drinking.

Weeks back, I made an appointment over the phone with a nutritionist, and her response was, 'Come and see me, and bring with you a journal of everything you put into your body over the next seven days in terms of food and drinks.' I completed this task, but like a true slouch, I cancelled my appointment thinking, 'What do I really need a nutritionist for anyway?'

But, for the purpose of my mission, I wrote down everything I put into my body for one week. And this is what it looked like:

Breakfast

The chart below shows my breakfast eating for the week:

	Breakfast	
	Food	Drinks
Monday	-	Red Bull
Tuesday	-	Red Bull
Wednesday	-	Red Bull
Thursday	Bacon/egg sandwich on white bread	Red Bull
Friday		Red Bull
Saturday	Belgian waffle with butter/maple syrup, two eggs	Red Bull / Orange juice
Sunday		Water

This chart looks incomplete. It's not. It's just that I am too lazy and unmotivated to eat breakfast. My thought pattern is 'I don't need breakfast.'

When I look at my breakfast consumption throughout the week, only one word comes to mind: embarrassing. And this is how I typically start my day – with no food. No brain food, no energy for a workout and no fuel to start my day, except for an energy drink. Apart from a bacon and egg sandwich coated with tomato sauce on the way home from a morning run along with my hangover cure of a Belgian waffle with a side of eggs, I normally go the morning with zero food. Fruit? None. Breakfast cereal? None. Brown bread with avocado? None. Is breakfast necessary? Yes!

According to Debra Wein, President of Sensible Nutrition[i]:

1 *Breakfast can improve your overall health. Research shows that individuals who consume breakfast every day report better mental and physical health than those who consume breakfast less frequently. In addition, individuals who consume breakfast regularly have a healthier lifestyle than non-breakfast eaters. Breakfasters are less likely to be smokers, drink less alcohol, and have a healthier diet.*

2 *Breakfast can keep you alert.*

i Wein, Debra (MS, RD, LDN www.sensiblenutrition.com), 2004, 'Breaking Ground with Breakfast', excerpt from Volume 3 #6 issue of National Strength and Conditioning Association Online Performance Journal <http://www.nsca-lift.org/perform/issues/0306.pdf>.

3 *Breakfast can help you emotionally.*
4 *Breakfast can enhance your mental performance.*
5 *The right breakfast can help you manage your weight.*
6 *Breakfast can enhance the overall quality of your diet.*

Along with these findings, it is simple common sense that eating breakfast starts my body's metabolism and gives me the fuel I need to start my mind and body for a 15-hour day. Simply put – it is essential. Yet, in looking at my own habits, three things strike me when I look at my breakfast consumption:

a It is non-existent;
b When consumption does exist, it is neither healthy nor balanced; and
c And because of a) and b) I am actually malnourished to start each day.

As for the excessive energy drink consumption, well this is a perfect example of where I have *no* idea of the contents of the food and drink I am consuming. 'It is an energy drink, therefore it must be healthy,' I assume. But now, in looking at the ingredients, my thoughts are 'what in the hell is taurine? Or Niacin? And why am I putting these things into my body?'

In fact, energy drinks have numerous ingredients in each can, all of which I have *no idea* about: taurine, glucuronolactone, cyanocobalamine, riboflavin, pyridoxide HCl, pantothenic acid, niacin and loads of caffeine and sugar. If that's not scary enough, some of this stuff is actually legally banned for consumption in some countries. And this is how I start my day? Something has to change!

Lunch

	Lunch	
	Food	Drinks
Monday	Chicken, mushroom, bacon crepe with a crème sauce	600ml Soft drink
Tuesday	Chicken laksa	600ml Soft drink
Wednesday	Low fat roasted chicken sandwich	Fresh fruit juice
Thursday	Asian diced, fried chicken on white rice topped with red curry sauce	Water
Friday	Greek salad with grilled chicken	Glass of white wine
Saturday	Sushi – raw tuna, salmon, and chicken/ avocado roll	Water
Sunday	Fish and chips with tartare sauce	600ml Soft drink

My lunch consumption can be categorised as salty takeaway food. Each day after my attempt at a gym run, I stop at the food court in the local mall, where I'm faced with endless lunch options. Chinese? Thai? Indian? Or a crepe? My decision comes from the sky; whatever I am feeling like, I buy. I do not listen to what my body needs, so health and nutrition is entirely neglected. While my chart shows some salad and fruit juice consumption, this comes mainly from guilt, rather than a conscious plan to eat well.

Dinner and Drinks

	Dinner	
	Food	Drinks
Monday	BBQ chicken, stuffing, and a salad with tomato, avocado, cheese and ranch dressing	2 Glasses of red wine
Tuesday	7 Layer Mexican dip, 3 chicken tacos with cheese & guacamole, and one slice of chocolate cake	2 Bottles of beer
Wednesday	$5 steak and mash at the pub	1 Bottle of white wine
Thursday	Chicken pad Thai, four Thai fried chicken wings	7 Schooners of beer
Friday	Garden Salad, 7 pieces of assorted pizza	6 Glasses of red wine, 1 vodka martini, 2 rum and colas and 2 tequila shots
Saturday	Brie with biscuits, 2 helpings of mushroom risotto, cookies 'n cream ice cream	2 bottles of red wine
Sunday	½ wheel of brie/biscuits, small portion of mushroom risotto, and ½ log of garlic bread	600ml Soft drink

The chart shows me how bad my nutrition intake is. I am so glad I didn't show up to the nutritionist bearing this!

I understand where my problem lies. I am a truly a flavour freak. Be it cooking for myself or ordering at a restaurant, my order is *never* based on nutritional value but *only* on the flavour that I feel like at the time; and, of course, with that usually comes an obscenely high amount of fat.

Having grown up in Dad's restaurant in Chicago, food was always a large part of my family's lifestyle, from weeknight meals to our holiday gatherings. I have always associated food with pleasure rather than having an understanding of its link with nutrition. Of course, along with my love for pleasure eating comes pleasure drinking.

I can see from my food chart that my weekly alcohol consumption is teetering *out of control*. I started as a Friday/Saturday drinker during my high school years, to become the drinks-anytime-anywhere-with-anybody type of lifestyle that I am immersed in today. And then, the vicious cycle starts – heaps of drinking leads to the big hangovers, which leads to demotivation at work or in the gym, which leads to feeding that hangover with bad food, which then leads to some serious weight gain and bad health. It's an ugly, deviant cycle.

Snacks

	Daily Snacks
Monday	Candy bar, apple
Tuesday	–
Wednesday	¾ packet of crisps
Thursday	¼ packet of crisps, banana
Friday	Aussie pie
Saturday	3 chocolate chip cookies
Sunday	Ice cream bar

Thankfully this is the last category to analyse, because by this point in time, I am truly grossed out by my consumption of crap. My snacks follow the same pattern as the other meals: high fat, high sodium, highly processed and loaded with sugar. Some of my snacks are daytime niceties, and some snacks are drunken post-bar feeds. Either way, I look at my consumption, and I don't need to be a nutritionist to know that my snacks have little-to-zero nutritional value.

From breakfast to dinner to the snacks in between, I look at my eating habits, and I can only think 'what in the world am I putting in my body?' Eating poorly has become instinctive for me. Put a labrador in water, and it will swim. Put me in a fast food restaurant and I will eat until food coma kicks in. But still, knowing that you eat and drink poorly is one thing - seeing it on paper? It is very powerful to actually see what poor habits I have developed and what a disservice I am doing to my health.

My Workouts

I regularly go to the gym. The problem is, most days I leave hardly breaking a sweat. My typical pattern during a gym day looks like this:

1. Enter gym with hangover.
2. Throw gear in locker.
3. Give serious thought to what deviant lunch choice I will make at the mall.
4. Walk over for a 15-second stretch with zero purpose except to have a perve and see who's around and who's looking good.
5. Head over to the treadmill where I'll run for 12 minutes or until I feel the full effects of my hangover, and stop.
6. Narrow down my deviant lunch options.
7. Back to the stretching area for the fastest abs workout in history.
8. Perve again.
9. Hit the shower.
10. Leave gym and head for a fatty, hangover-cure type of lunch.

What a sad situation and a cycle that I repeat way too often. And what is missing in my gym day? A fitness plan! A goal! A reason for being there! It's almost as if I believe in magic, and with that the swipe of my gym card and my physical presence alone, magically my love-handles will disappear and in their place a buff gym guy will appear.

In my mind, I think I believe that my effort at the gym is negating the prior night's drinks and bad food. But deep down I know (and can see) that bad health is winning. Working out is meant to make you feel good, feel healthy and make you fit – yet I consistently feel like shit and hate the way I look in the mirror. I am not happy at all, yet I cannot seem to make a change for the good.

My Body

Because of my bad workouts, my alcohol consumption and my poor eating this is how I look:

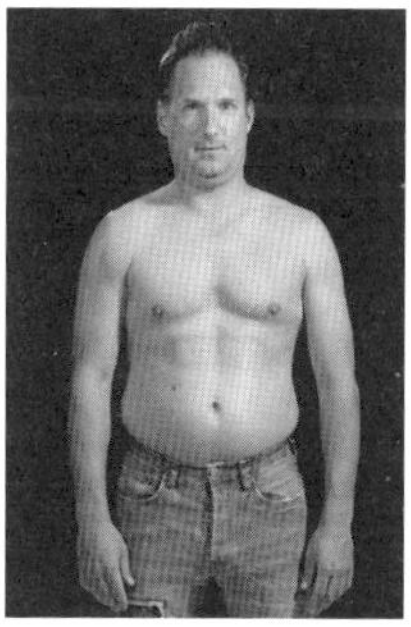

This photo sickens me. It's shocking and hard to look at, but, let's face it, it's me. And if the obesity rate in Australia is at or over 60 per cent, then this is how too many of us look. To see myself looking so mentally melancholy and so physically soft – it is truly alarming.

At this point I weigh 88kgs, which is the heaviest I've been in ages. My body fat is way too high at 27.5 per cent, and for the life of me I just don't know why I let myself get like this. It just seemed to happen as the days went by.

When I relax my body, as I did in the photo, I have a beer belly that only guys in beer commercials should own. Although waist measurement seems to be the proxy by which we judge our weight loss and weight gain, I really want to rid myself of this embarrassingly enormous gut. I take a circumference measurement of the fattest part of my gut – right at the belly button area. But when I try, the 101-centimetre (40-inch) tape measure won't even reach all the way around my belly. You know you're in a bad state when the tape measure used to measure your couch won't fit around your waist. It turns out that my belly is around 112 centimetres (44-inches) around, and my waist size is at 91 centimetres (36 inches).

For me, however, it isn't so much about numbers and what I would like them to be; instead, I just want to have that fit, healthy shape that you see on people who look after themselves.

My belly to waist ratio – or as I will call it, my *cir-gut-ference ratio* – is 44:36 or 1.22. The statistics, which must change are:

	Day 0
Weight	88
Body Fat	27.50%
Belly Button Circumference	44
Jeans Size	36
Cir-gut-ference Difference	1.22

I really shouldn't be surprised by the numbers, because I know I am deeply embedded in an abusive life, where I am not caring for my body, but am instead abusing my system with horrible food and way too much alcohol. The photo and the statistics are mere indicators of my lifestyle.

3

Telling it Like it Is

I'm in a rut…a deep one. I don't need a doctor or a personal trainer to tell me my situation because I have seen it on paper and I am honest enough with myself to know where I am at, health-wise. *I am a chubby-arse who needs to make a change*.

So this is where my story of improved health begins, although I am not quite sure where it will end. I am not a personal trainer, I am not a nutritionist and I am not a doctor; hell, I'm not even a writer! But I am a chubby chap who needs to make a lifestyle change.

I know that somewhere deep, down below those love handles and insecurities, I have the strength to make this change. And on some level, I think that if I succeed in my journey, then maybe my words, my challenges and whatever plan I follow can be used to help others.

Now, I am not taking the high road and becoming an overnight authority on health and proclaiming 'What is good for me is therefore good for all,' but as up to 60 per cent of us are obese, chances are we all are guilty of living in the same manner, with the same poor habits and with the same bulging waistline, because:

- We're eating the same crappy food, with the same crappy ingredients, with little regard for our health;
- We're drinking too much alcohol; and
- We're not getting proper exercise.

Oh, I know it's a bit more complex than this, but the observation is quite simple – there are so many of us who are not looking after our bodies, our minds and our health, and it's time for our group in society to make a change. We need to stop immediately with the bullshit excuses of why we haven't done this…and start living life the way it was meant to be.

Unfortunately, I don't think too many in our obese culture are *telling it like it is*, and instead of being completely honest with ourselves, I think we are creating our own Obesity Snowball.

The Obesity Snowball

My abusive lifestyle has contributed to and created an *Obesity Snowball*. A snowball that travels downhill collects more snow, grows larger, keeps travelling downward, and it doesn't stop until something makes it stop.

My abusive lifestyle and poor health is no different. I am somewhere in the middle of my downhill slide, feeling like trash mentally, yet I continue to feed myself more junk, drink more alcohol, and so my downward slide towards even poorer health is perpetuated.

So many of us have just settled into our lifestyle, become lazy and accepted that we are fat, and that there is no way around it. And when that vicious cycle of *eating, getting fat, comfort eating to feel better, then getting fatter* starts, well, our Obesity Snowball just gains more momentum and keeps on rolling.

However, the beauty in being human, as opposed to being a snowball, is that we have the mental capacity to stop that momentum. We *can* say no at anytime.

The Doctor Dilemma

We have scientists galore to help advise and create a plan to fix the environment – so why can't doctors who deal with our health help us with our obesity challenge?

Doctors are fantastic. I respect their education, I respect their knowledge and I respect their compassion to help people get well. I also respect the difficulty that their job entails when telling a weeping family that their son or daughter won't survive the night. The doctor-patient relationship is a difficult one, and I think the secret of good doctors is that they try to create an open yet comforting relationship with their patients.

A doctor is certainly there to aid us, but if I take a look from another angle, that doctor is also a business unit that needs to make money to survive. That business unit is supported by patients, otherwise known as consumers. And for that business to be successful, it must make its consumers – who come in feeling nervous, insecure and vulnerable – leave feeling comfortable and relaxed. Why? So those patients will be return customers the next time they are unwell and that business will grow and make more money.

But by making patients 'comfortable', the strength and urgency in the obesity health message is getting lost. Because, I know that a doctor would say to me...

> *Mike, you know you have a couple of extra pounds on you there that you could probably lose.*

What that doctor really should be saying is...

> *Your health is in a state of shit. You are overweight, and you are staring diabetes, heart problems, back problems, liver issues, bad ankles and knees right in the face. Oh, and forget about having a glass of wine with your grandchildren – you'll never make it at the pace you're going. Either make a change in your lifestyle or severe medical issues will do it for you.*

This is where the doctor dilemma lies. Do they tell it to us like it is? Or do they prefer to give it to us in a soft way ensuring we don't get too embarrassed, too insecure about our obese appearance? After all, a lot of internal problems are just that – internal and hidden. Obesity is an external, very personal appearance issue that we're already aware of as patients, and therefore doctors aren't as harsh about expressing the severity of it. Well, if doctors aren't going to do it, then we should at least be honest with ourselves.

Because if doctors aren't telling it like it is, giving us these *obese-comfort messages* over and over again, allowing the excess weight to stay where it is, the next message will be the rough one. It will be the 'You have diabetes' message, or the 'You had a massive heart attack' message. And then? It's too damn late to do anything about it.

So, I'm here to say it like it is – sometimes cursing like a sailor, sometimes not – but I assure you that my health, my plan and my journey to stop my Obesity Snowball and get fit and healthy will be an honest, open one.

4

Three Phases of Health

I will never claim to be a psychologist or the deepest of thinkers because, in the end, I am a chap who believes that simple problems require simple solutions.

But today, I had a few thoughts in the deeper end of the pool. I identified the three behaviours, the three phases that many of us tend to live in at some point or another. The first two of these phases are:

The Abuse Phase; and
The Control Phase.

The Abuse Phase

The Abuse Phase is where we don't watch what we eat, we drink too much, we don't go to the gym and as a result we are filling up hospitals with obesity-related diseases. Our Obesity Snowballs are rolling downhill quickly, and our abusive health behaviour is being passed down to our children, where the cycle continues into the next generation. With obesity levels around 60 per cent, it is probably fair to say that much of society is in that Abuse Phase.

We all know people who have smoked for sixty years of their lives, and somehow their bodies have coped with it. They might look like hell, with their skin, their eyes and their insides appearing in poor form, but somehow their bodies just keep on surviving. It amazes me how much abuse the body can cope with, and for a lot of us, this gives us the green light to just keep doing the same old thing. But is this truly living? Is coping in the Abuse Phase a fun way of life? Is it really where we want to be? I really don't think so.

The first stage to leaving this phase is to recognise you are living an abusive lifestyle. Secondly, it is necessary to understand where you want to go once you decide to stop abusing yourself – and that is to the Control Phase.

The Control Phase

I am confident that I have lost control of my health – so much so that I am not even sure I know what control is or what it would feel like to have it.

I imagine that people in the Control Phase know what's good and what's bad for their body; they don't overdo things, they are conscious of their mental and physical wellbeing, and they have the power to direct and determine the direction of their health. They know there are cheeky choices at the grocery store and at the pub, yet they choose wisely.

Sounds ideal, right? I think if I was in the Control Phase I could be that fit guy who enjoys the outdoors, enjoys a long run, has that body confidence yet still enjoys a few beers and a nice meal after a long week. I want to be that guy who can enjoy a pizza knowing the next day he will be at the gym to work it off, so no harm's done.

And later in life? I want to be half of that 70-year old couple who still goes for long walks, holding hands. I want to be able to still enjoy a nice meal with my wife while drinking a toast with a beautiful glass of Hunter Valley Shiraz. These people are truly in *control*. They know that a healthy life is all about balance. They still enjoy the occasional naughty pleasures in life, but they balance it with health and moderation to always live a life that is physically and mentally balanced.

So, with so many of us living in the Abuse Phase, but wanting to jump into the Control Phase, the question is: How in the hell do I get access to the Control Phase? Well, that is where the challenge may lie, and that is why the third phase exists – the Change Phase.

The Change Phase

I wish I could wake up one day and just erase all my bad habits and have them magically replaced with good ones. Sometimes I think I can actually do that, when once a month, after a binge weekend, I wake up on Monday morning, feeling as fat and shitty as I can possibly feel, and I have that super healthy Monday, thinking I am off to a new, fresh start that will last forever. But, of course, by Tuesday, all it takes is a pizza commercial, or a mate to put the callout for a social drink and I am right back into my old lifestyle.

We often live 100 per cent in the Abuse Phase, yet we think that by cutting out 10 per cent of our naughty behaviour, we can turn our entire wellbeing around. But think about it: a thief who makes a promise to steal less is still a thief, and a smoker who goes from 20mg cigarettes to 10mg cigarettes is still a smoker. So to be living in the Abuse Phase and to decide to abuse my body less makes no sense, and is definitely not the answer to my problem. Less unhealthy does not mean healthy.

In order to go from the Abuse Phase to the Control Phase, a giant step needs to be taken.

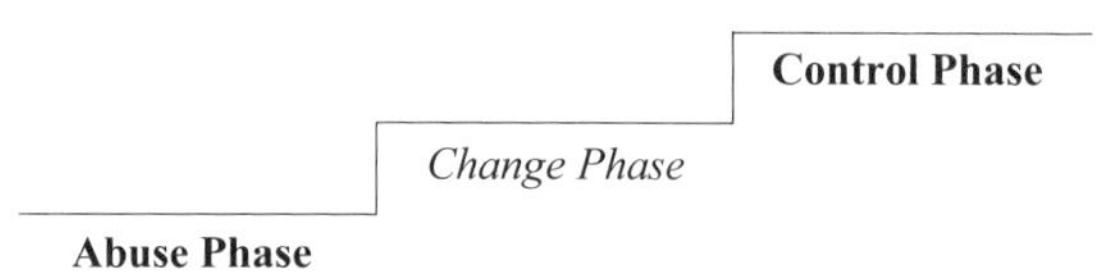

It's a simple depiction, but the steps above illustrate the simple point that from the Abuse Phase, we must step into the Change Phase before reaching the Control Phase. And, sadly, there is no skipping any steps to reach the Control Phase.

Within the Change Phase, I need to ensure there are healthy, fresh meals, simple, efficient workouts and no alcohol. I will be in the Change Phase when I am living a clean and healthy life. And once those days become instinctive? Well, then, and only then, will I be (hopefully) ready to graduate into the Control Phase.

The Control Phase is where I will be a happier person, both emotionally and physically. Mates call me the jolly drinker and happy eater, and at gatherings I am chatty, social and always having a great time. But deep down I have stopped to think about my health and know I reside in the Abuse Phase. When I'm home, and when I'm alone, I know the state I am in is not a good one, and with my 35th birthday fast approaching, it is actually a really crappy and depressing place to be.

5

How Did I Get This Way?

What in the hell happened to me?

When I was younger, I was out each day playing basketball, baseball, football, golf… everything and anything to be active. But when you're young, you have endless energy, no muscle soreness and all the time in the world to be outdoors and active. But then along came university and working years, and, well, the basketball games stopped, the drinking nights began and those healthy meals that Mum cooked up somehow got replaced by my own unhealthy cooking and takeaway meals, and hence, I went from a high school athlete to a current day *fathlete*.

I Stopped Thinking

In trying to determine where I went wrong, I could make all the same and lame excuses, but the truth is:

I simply stopped thinking.

I know it sounds simplistic, but it's true. When it came to food and my health, I stopped thinking.

I believe there are two types of eaters – thinkers and reactors. The thinkers give some thought to their intake, they think about their weekly eating and, although they still have a cheeky night out with fish and chips or pizza on the menu, they know the effect it has on their body, so they also balance it out with subsequent meals of fresh veggies, fruit and fish, and a regular exercise regime.

Unfortunately, I am from the other camp of eaters – the reactors. If I see food that looks good, regardless of fat or sugar content, or the health benefits (or lack thereof), my reaction is to eat it. I don't give any thought to an eating plan or which foods are good for my heart, my muscles or my energy levels. Instead, I just think about how fantastic it would taste, and before the thought pattern is finished, I've usually already eaten it. And, of course, reactors usually opt for portion sizes that mirror their shirt size: extra large!

It is this very train of thought that adds those excess kilograms.

I Stopped Listening to My Body

Our bodies speak to us, but if we don't listen we can never actually be healthy. Think about it:

a When your body is in a poor state of health, like mine, toilet time is hot, wet and fast – that is, if you actually ever go to the toilet! This is our body's way of telling us that it doesn't like what we are putting into its digestive system, and usually it's talking pretty loudly, but do we actually hear what it's saying to us?

b We climb two flights of stairs, yet we are breathing like we have just summitted Mount Everest! After small bursts of activity, oxygen is on short supply, and this is our body's way of telling us that we need to get to the gym and improve our fitness!

c Too many days start with a hangover, which is our brain's way of telling us it does not like the overload of alcoholic chemicals we have consumed.

Bad toilet time, breathing difficulties and a big hangover are all the ways our body is telling us we're not doing right by it. Yet, even though I know it all, why do I consistently wake up hung over, skip the gym and go eat more junk food?

Because rather than listening to what my body is telling me, I have refused to take the hint, and health-wise I am digging a deep, body-abusive hole for myself that I need to crawl out of.

Excuse Syndromes

Excuses never run short when it comes to my health. Here are a few of my most used, which many folks have probably heard come out of their mouths, once or twice!

The *First* Syndrome

I can't even count how many times I've said 'I'll just have one more big weekend, and then I'll start my health plan on the first.' I think that a new month or a new year is, psychologically, the best day to make a fresh, healthy start. But, in all honesty, it's probably just so I can continue binging on the bad stuff for a bit longer.

And, of course, when that date does arrive, I find another excuse to avoid making the change, so I never actually end up creating or starting that health and workout plan and instead, I just fall straight back into the same detrimental patterns.

The Government Syndrome

In the past few years, I've noticed quite a disturbing trend. The news, the newspapers, they're all saying it. I hear things like:

> *The government needs to do something about obesity...*
> *The fast-food restaurants need to be banned from commercials...*

This is all complete bullshit. When I want something, I go and get it. I pay for it. And then I consume it. The key word there is *I*. Are we such babies that we need the government to create signs like those explicit signs we find on cigarette packets, that might say:

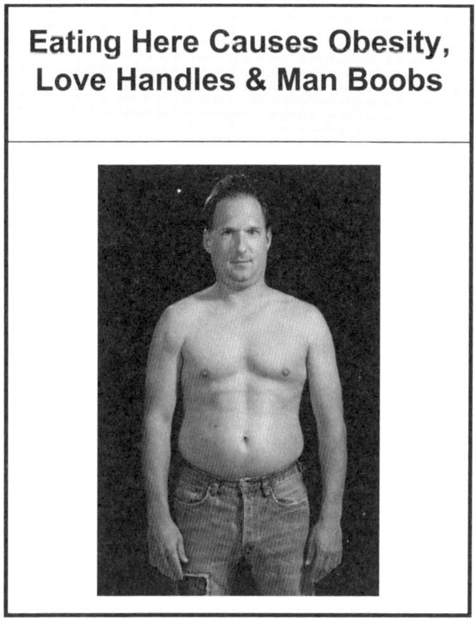

It sucks when I realise that such a sign would actually work! Of course, it sucks even more when I look at that sign and know I have the ideal physique to spearhead such a campaign!

Obesity isn't about governments, and it isn't about corporate fast food joints. It's about me. It's about what I put in my refrigerator and what I cook in my kitchen. It's about my choices and what I decide to put into my body. It's time to stop waiting for governments to institute mediocre changes and think about myself and the changes *I* need to make in order to get myself healthy.

The Oprah Syndrome

It's not uncommon to hear women say 'If I had a billion dollars, I'd have me a personal trainer and a personal chef and I'd be skinny, just like Oprah!'

Well, I say 'bullshit' to that! Oprah is a billionaire, having built a business empire, and having worked tirelessly for so long. If anybody has an excuse to comfort eat, workout less and sleep more, it's Oprah Winfrey! Yet even billionaires have to put on their gym clothes, hit the treadmill and sweat off the fat like us mere mortals. How do I know? My brother has seen her at his gym in Chicago and she goes through all the hard yards to sweat it out, just like the rest of us!

The *It's In My Genes* Syndrome

Some people say, 'Both my mum and dad are big, and that's why I'm big too. It's in my genes to be this size; there's really nothing I can do about it.'

Nice excuse, but it's wrong.

The truth is that mum and dad are big because they did not eat healthy foods, and they did not exercise. You are also big because you, as a child, ate what they ate. It's not your genes, it's the lack of exercise and nutrition they handed down to you.

The *I have no time* Syndrome

I've said it, and I'm sick of hearing myself say it – *I have no time*.

Enough is enough. I must find the time or make the time. It's my life, it's my health. And it's my decision to be in the body I am in. It really is that simple.

If my body, my life and my health are in a state of crisis, shouldn't I find the time to do everything I can in order to make a healthy change?

To reiterate this a little more poetically and philosophically:

> *A man too busy to take care of his health is like a mechanic too busy to take care of his tools.*
>
> *Spanish Proverb*

The *I've tried everything and nothing works for me* Syndrome

I love this one. We have all tried the fad diets, the fad diet pills, and bought all the 1-800 workout gizmos, just so that we can conclude nothing works for us. But have we actually tried eating healthy and exercising regularly? It's common sense for us all, and it's actually the only strategy that is guaranteed to work.

I know that in order to change my body and change my life I have to dump all the excuses and shed all of those excuse syndromes. Therefore, I will make this declaration right here, right now. I will now turn every 'I can't' into 'I will.'

> *I will get healthy, I will make a positive change, and I will turn my life around.*

I am going to find a workout plan that is about what I *can* do and what I *can* eat, because the excuses have gotten me absolutely nowhere so far.

Time to Make a Change

In a small town in Georgia, USA lies a bar called Mulligan's which serves a dish they call *The Hamdog*. The Hamdog consists of a hot dog wrapped in a beef patty that is deep fried, covered with chilli, cheese and onions, and served on a hoagie bun topped with a fried egg and two fistfuls of fries.

If you have ever consumed a Hamdog, or the thought of consuming one makes your mouth water with delight, then you are like me, and – chances are – it is time to make some changes in *your* lifestyle too!

Do you have any of these signs in your life?

a The 'Elevator is out, please use stairs' sign at work sends you into a John McEnroe-esque string of expletives, and you only work on the second floor.

b You rip the tag off the back of your Levi's because you see no reason why your waist size should be advertised like a billboard on your arse.

- **c** You reach the front of the queue and the Qantas ticketing agent looks you over and suggests you buy two seats.
- **d** You start to accept the email newsletters from the National Association to Advance Fat Acceptance. (Yes, there is a group in the US by that name!)
- **e** On your approach to a barbeque, the sight of a vacant wicker chair at a friend's outdoor patio has you thinking, 'Uh-oh, that may not hold.'
- **f** Seven days a week you look at your watch and declare that it's 'beer o'clock.'
- **g** You've woken up at 4am, to find yourself fully naked on your living room floor next to a half eaten, foot-long meatball and cheese sub sandwich. (Yes, I have done this.)

If you answered yes to any of these, or have had similar experiences, then join me in making this commitment to change.

It will be damn difficult. We are stuck in the same pattern, with the same habits, and it will be hard for us to break those patterns. But we must either stop our gluttonous lifestyles now, or we will allow obesity-related diseases to stop our lives altogether.

Now is the time to embrace change, to start *thinking* in a healthy manner, and to start *listening* to the language our body is speaking.

Now is the time to embrace change.

Setting a Goal

I see movies, television and gossip magazines and think 'I want to have *his* body,' where the 'his' I refer to is usually a millionaire actor or athlete with the most glamorous, glorious body the world has ever seen. So, my follow-up thought is usually pretty quick to emerge, and it usually sounds something like, 'Well, his body is unattainable, so you might as well pass me another beer and some more chips.' I do not believe I can attain the unattainable and, therefore, I simply don't try.

In order for me to achieve a physical and mental change, I will retrain my thoughts and reassess my goals, so that they are always simple and obtainable.

Have a Physical Goal

For example, while I would love to have the muscular arms of an AFL player, a chiselled face, fit and muscular legs, and six-pack abs, the reality is that a four-pack with a little bag of ice hanging around at the bottom would be a decent second place, in my mind; so, I need to keep my goals real. I mean, I'm fresh from wiping the fried chicken off my hands that I ate for lunch, so in order for me to have a shot at being successful at this, it's probably best I think a little bit more realistically about where I would like to head, rather than set the bar too high to begin with.

So, here it is:

> *I want to look good in jeans and a t-shirt, and I want to feel comfortable at the beach wearing a pair of shorts and no shirt.*

Why jeans and a t-shirt? Because for me, that is the most simple way of displaying my body. Now, I know that women the world over spend hundreds and thousands on fashionable dresses, jewellery and make-up, but in my opinion, throw a girl in a nice pair of jeans with a tight fitting t-shirt and you've got the sexiest outfit one can wear!

The jeans and t-shirt ensemble is all about exposing the true me; there is no hiding behind double breasted suit jackets, untucked collared shirts, or bulky jumpers. It's just me, a pair of jeans and a t-shirt, and if I can look good in that – then, in my mind, I will have succeeded in my journey.

So how much weight do I need to lose to get there? At 88kgs, maybe eight or ten kilograms is a reasonable goal? I'm heading into unchartered waters, so I really don't know. You wouldn't predict how much gold you are going to collect if you have never sifted for it before, so because I don't really know how my body will respond to good workouts and healthy eating, I will not put a number on the unknown.

What I do know is that I want to see myself in pictures looking *shit hot* in jeans and a t-shirt. Because the image burned into my brain of my topless photo with my love handles and man boobs – well, that has to be erased from my memory somehow!

Set a Mental Goal

At the moment, I lack confidence and motivation, and I know this is directly related to how I feel about my body, as well a result of all the junk I am eating each day.

So, my mental goal is:

> *I want the satisfaction of making a change. I don't want to quit and I want to enjoy living a new, healthy lifestyle. I want a clear, hangover-free head, and I want to feel secure about my body. And at the end of my journey, I want to take a deep breath and be able to look myself in the mirror and say, 'I did it, and now I have a new life.'*

Depressed but Time to Move On

There are a tonne of 'I wish' moments going on in my life. I wish I looked better, I wish I was slimmer, I wish I was healthier, I wish I ate better and I wish I felt better about myself overall. It kind of all snowballs to make me feel, well, less than average. But those feelings of depression and gloom are stopping right *now*.

Sure, it's easier said than done, but if this is a step towards making a change in my lifestyle, then I will commit to getting it done. I know I have the tools within to pull myself out of my mental slump, because I learned how from my dad.

My father survived numerous bouts of illness throughout his life, including pneumonia and spinal meningitis. Too many surgeries caused the spinal fluid in his back to turn him into a paraplegic, confined to a wheelchair. But, despite his condition, he never let anything stop him from doing what he wanted – from driving a car, to becoming a successful restaurateur. I'm sure he felt limited, at times, but he never complained about his situation nor did he ever mention the intensity of his chronic pain.

My parents were divorced, and over the years my dad moved from being *just* my dad to being my friend. He was somebody to talk to every day about everything, from the deeper things in life to the superficial day-to-day gossip. He used to meet me in downtown Chicago for swanky two-and-a-half hour meals where we would bullshit over a few bottles of wine, and just hang out.

In September of 1996 my dad's health took a turn for the worse. I don't know if it was my denial of his declining health, or the fact he'd always recovered after being so sick so often and back working at the restaurant, but I just never entertained the thought that he might not make it; I didn't believe it was possible. Unfortunately, that day came when the impossible did happen.

The first person to arrive at my father's wake was someone I will never forget. He had recently lost his own father, and he told me, 'Remember this day. Because the day that you lose your father is the day that you will never be the same person again. Today, you don't know how this will affect you, but it will and you will be changed forever.'

At the time, I didn't really know what to think of this, but he was right. My dad passed away, and it was the most difficult, testing, awful, horrible time of my life. It is impossible to describe the loss of a parent to someone who hasn't experienced it for themselves. For me, even though I'm an adult, my mum and dad always provided a sort of psychological *safety net*, where I knew they would be there if I ever needed them. So, when one of them is gone, that safety net disappears, and the hole that is left behind cannot be filled by anything or anyone; it's simply left vacant forever and, as a result, you are changed, emotionally, forever.

With tragedy comes perspective. When I was younger, I would get so stressed about the little things; from my team losing a game, to having to work overtime – all sorts of minor issues could set me off. But after losing my father, I truly understood what was important, and I developed a healthier outlook on life. I no longer dwelled on disappointment for days on end, and I adopted the approach of 'have a cry or a whinge if you need it, but when the next day arrives, get the fuck over it and move on.'

So I am going to take this exact approach with my current state of health. I am done dwelling on my poor health, my love handles and my Michelin Man-like shape. Tonight is the last time I will whinge. Tomorrow I am waking up and taking up residence on the path to making a change.

My goal is ambitious yet realistic, and I finally feel I'm in the right mindset to make a change – I want to get my life and my health back, and now I just need the right plan to help me get there.

6

The City Caveman Plan

The Search for an Answer

All over the world, the health industry is filled with empty promises and products that over-promise and under-deliver in their health solutions. Fitness and health have become so complex, with so many options and so many 'schemes', I simply didn't know where to start.

My options for a diet or a workout plan were limitless. I could shop at health food shops, vitamin centres, or weight-lifting superstores. I could sign up at a weight loss centre, get a personal trainer, or skip it all and see a plastic surgeon. Everybody, everywhere claims to have a plan that works, for quite a pretty price.

However, the thought hit me one day in the shower: what would happen if I bucked the trend of all this futuristic, scientific shit, and went back to the very basics by eating fresh and healthy food like the cavemen did? And what if I went to the gym and just did simple, no-frills, one-hour workouts?

And that was the beginning of the City Caveman Plan.

Meeting Annie Clark

We all have to realise our personal shortcomings, and when it comes to fitness, I realise that I am not a personal trainer, I am a chubby drinker! So, in order to expand on the concept of the City Caveman Plan, I met with personal trainers to source some ideas, feedback and perhaps a potential partner who could help me during my journey to regain my health and life.

I met up with quite a few trainers; some thought my Caveman idea was ridiculous, some charged $100 just to meet up with me, some recommended I eat only raw food, some didn't 'walk their talk' and some were so Hulk-like strong that I couldn't imagine them identifying with my situation, or the place where I wanted to be, either physically or mentally.

What I noticed most from these meetings, was that so many personal trainers focus on the physical aspects of health. Sure, I want to change my body, and they might be able to provide one hour of training each day to help me do so, but what about the other twenty-three hours in the day? What about the mental difficulties I would encounter in making such drastic changes? I did find it quite challenging to find a trainer who had the smarts, sensitivity and understanding to train me and provide me with the emotional support needed to actually change my lifestyle.

That is, until I met with Annie Clark.

I met Annie for lunch, and what I immediately liked about her was her succinctness. There were no long, lengthy, bullshit answers. She had a simple, direct, healthy approach to life and fitness. She could understand my life of debauchery, but she also knew the way to health was to cut out all the shit. Annie Clark is a Personal Trainer, Psychologist, fitness competitor, and mother. She has been involved in the fitness industry for 18 years and has won numerous fitness competitions within Australia. I needed lifestyle advice, and Annie was just the professional to give it to me.

I confessed to Annie the contents of my eating diary, with the pizza, the drinks and all the junk I put into my body. I told her that I didn't want to look like Arnold Schwarzenegger, but that I just wanted to gain mind and body confidence, and that I wanted to feel comfortable at the beach, and look great in jeans and a t-shirt.

I told her that I would keep a daily diary of what was going through my mind, my workouts, and the emotional ups and downs, so that she could track my progress, and when I asked Annie what she thought of the concept of eating healthy, fresh and tasty foods, combined with a simple but regular exercise program (i.e., the City Caveman Plan), her response was, 'Yeah, let's do this.'

And so we did.

City Caveman Eating Plan: The 10-10-10 Fat Rule

The Caveman Eating Plan is about consuming lots of fresh fruit and vegetables, and lean sources of protein, such as grilled fish. It allows for nutritious, healthy, balanced and tasty meals to be eaten which are all low in fat, sugar and salt, but high in nutrients.

It aims to reduce the daily fat intake per meal to 10 grams at breakfast, 10 grams at lunch and 10 grams at dinner.

I have been taking in around 100 grams of fat per day, which is completely insane because it is affecting my workouts and my waistline big time!

I agreed to the 10-10-10 rule but soon realised that I actually had little idea what a meal or snack containing 10 grams of fat looked like. I had never grabbed anything off the shelves and spun it around to look at the nutritional contents so, with the aid of Google, I found a few well-known items and their fat contents:

Item	Fat Grams
Double Cheeseburger	33
Big Serving of Crisps	15
Cheesecake	18
Deep Dish Cheese	100

I quickly learned that some of my old favourites would definitely not be fitting into the Caveman 10-10-10 eating plan. So long, Mr Pringles.

In order to achieve the 10-10-10 rule, I would have to 'strip' my food down to basics. So rather than a typical meal of fish and chips, I need to strip out the frying and replace it with grilling, and I need to swap the fried potatoes with boiled potatoes. This alone would save me 50 to 60 grams of fat in just one meal. Alcohol and sugary soft drinks are out, and they are to be replaced with water and freshly squeezed juices. I need to start thinking of food as both a nutritional and energy source for everyday activities and workouts, rather than viewing food as an activity or for comfort eating.

The City Caveman Eating Plan says I must:

a have a healthy breakfast;

b eat only fresh food (and when unsure, ask myself, 'Would a Caveman eat it like that?');

c grill, rather than deep fry;

d eat nothing that contains additives, preservatives or colourings;

e consume only meals that contain no more than 10 grams of fat;

f use spices, not salt, to add flavour;

g not consume alcohol; and,

h drink 2 to 3 litres of water every day.

Now, I will not be heading down the organic-only path. For me, the thought of having to find organic food is an added stress, not to mention the increased costs to do so. In my mind, a tomato is a tomato and a banana is a banana. So, no organics for me for now. And no eating birdseed or tofu burgers either; this is simply not an option for me or my taste buds. The Plan needs to be realistic and simple; otherwise I know I won't stick to it.

The City Caveman Plan will never be a *diet* because I simply love to eat! I've always thought that diets are for fools because they simply don't work. Dieting always seems to be equated with going without, or going hungry, and I am determined to feed myself, feel full and still enjoy the taste of healthy meals while on this Plan. So, I won't diet, but I *can* take on the City Caveman Plan, which will hopefully change my eating patterns for the better.

City Caveman Workout Plan

Workouts prescribed in reality television shows that are big hits in the TV ratings are unrealistic, and sometimes even dangerous, for the average person. Annie would never prescribe such intense, long workouts for me because, like the Eating Plan, the Workout Plan also needs to be achievable, realistic and simple so that I will stick to it.

I told Annie that I would not be running around the gym like a goof. I told her that due to insecurities about my body, I did not want to have to do wacky exercises that draw attention to me at the gym. So, we decided that the City Caveman Plan workouts should be comprised of six simple workouts per week, each lasting no longer than one hour.

The weight training routine would work the entire body and would be broken down into three days. Day 1 is for training the shoulders, biceps and triceps; Day 3 is for the legs; and Day 5 for the chest and back. Each of these programs will be 20 minutes in duration, in addition to 20 minutes of cardio training. Then, on the days in between I will undertake forty minutes of cardiovascular activities, such as walking, running, biking, swimming, etc.

I also want to improve my abs, so on the cardio training days I will also work my abdominal muscles, using a simple training program that John, my brother in Chicago, recommended. He's lean and fit, so his abdominal plan is the one I shall follow.

Page 50 contains the detailed City Caveman Workout Plan, but below is a summary of my weekly Caveman workouts:

	Weekly Workout Plan						
	Monday	**Tuesday**	**Wednesday**	**Thursday**	**Friday**	**Saturday**	**Sunday**
Cardio (40min)		X		X		X	
Abs		X		X		X	
Cardio (20min)	X		X		X		
Shoulders	X						
Triceps	X						
Biceps	X						
Chest					X		
Back					X		
Legs			X				

It feels pretty damn good to actually have a plan and a strategy to get my health back on track. But, deep down, I know that I am only 5 per cent of the way there, because while the answer is pretty simple and pretty easy, the process of executing this Plan and the process of change is not. *Change* is where the true challenge lies.

City Caveman Accountability

My weakness, my own Achilles heal is, unfortunately, myself. Any kind of workout plan that I have previously attempted has not been successful, largely because I've never held myself accountable for my results.

So, now that I have a formal plan, in the City Caveman Plan, I must build in some accountability measures to ensure I stay on track and so I can monitor my progress on a daily basis.

I own my belly, because I paid for all the shit that has gone in there, and so I feel like I need to take the steps to also claim ownership of my Workout Plan. The way I think is best to do this is to sign something that shows I, Mike Jarosky, made a commitment to a 40-day plan. My contract is below:

Caveman Contract

I, declare that I will abide by the Caveman Code of 40 days of:

- fresh, healthy eating;
- daily workouts as designed; and
- 2 litres of water per day.

I will avoid all processed foods, flavour enhanced items, fast food, soda drinks, and anything else that has made me chubby in the past. Pizza, brie, beers, late night Macca runs, chocolate, Aussie pies, and all other goodies that were not available during the caveman years will not be consumed for this 40 day period, while I get fit, healthy, and look better in my jeans/tshirt.

Signed: ____________________

Caveman Contract

Monday	Tuesday	Wednesday	Thursday	Friday	Saturday	Sunday
Food	Food	Food	Food	Food	Food	Food
5min JR, 20min cardio; Shoulder, Tri, Bi	40min cardio; 5min JR, abs	20min cardio; Legs	40min cardio; 5min JR, abs	5min JR, 20min cardio; Chest, Back	40min cardio; 5min JR, abs	
2 litres water	2 litres water	2 litres water	2 litres water	2 litres water	2 litres water	2 litres water
Food	Food	Food	Food	Food	Food	Food
5min JR, 20min cardio; Shoulder, Tri, Bi	40min cardio; 5min JR, abs	20min cardio; Legs	40min cardio; 5min JR, abs	5min JR, 20min cardio; Chest, Back	40min cardio; 5min JR, abs	
2 litres water	2 litres water	2 litres water	2 litres water	2 litres water	2 litres water	2 litres water
Food	Food	Food	Food	Food	Food	Food
5min JR, 20min cardio; Shoulder, Tri, Bi	40min cardio; 5min JR, abs	20min cardio; Legs	40min cardio; 5min JR, abs	5min JR, 20min cardio; Chest, Back	40min cardio; 5min JR, abs	
2 litres water	2 litres water	2 litres water	2 litres water	2 litres water	2 litres water	2 litres water
Food	Food	Food	Food	Food	Food	Food
5min JR, 20min cardio; Shoulder, Tri, Bi	40min cardio; 5min JR, abs	20min cardio; Legs	40min cardio; 5min JR, abs	5min JR, 20min cardio; Chest, Back	40min cardio; 5min JR, abs	
2 litres water	2 litres water	2 litres water	2 litres water	2 litres water	2 litres water	2 litres water
Food	Food	Food	Food	Food	Food	Food
5min JR, 20min cardio; Shoulder, Tri, Bi	40min cardio; 5min JR, abs	20min cardio; Legs	40min cardio; 5min JR, abs	5min JR, 20min cardio; Chest, Back	40min cardio; 5min JR, abs	
2 litres water	2 litres water	2 litres water	2 litres water	2 litres water	2 litres water	2 litres water
Food	Food	Food	Food	Food		
5min JR, 20min cardio; Shoulder, Tri, Bi	40min cardio; 5min JR, abs	20min cardio; Legs	40min cardio; 5min JR, abs	5min JR, 20min cardio; Chest, Back	Celebrate!!!	
2 litres water	2 litres water	2 litres water	2 litres water	2 litres water		

So, there it is. Upon signing it, I am committed and accountable to living a new lifestyle. I did feel a bit goofy when I sat down and created the Caveman Contract, but I really think it is a critical part of achieving success.

Now, I know I won't be taken to court and exposed on the news if I bow out at Day 12 but, deep down, I really do feel accountable for my actions. Now that it's on paper, I feel committed to not letting myself or Annie down.

With the Caveman Contract having such a distinct effect on my commitment to the Plan, I wanted something similar to illustrate my daily eating and workout progress, so I created an amendment to the Contract – a Daily Contract – so that I have a checklist to tick off each day that is centred around the Eating Plan, the Workout Plan and my water intake.

So, at the end of each day, when I follow my 10-10-10 eating plan I earn a tick in the food box. When I do the appropriate workout for the day, then I can tick the workout box. And if I consume my two to three litres of water per day, then that box will also be ticked.

For me, this Daily Contract is not like a test at university where 90 per cent is a great score and earns applause and praise. This is my health, and this is my life, so I am aiming to tick every box, every day.

I am going to tape my Daily Contract on my mirror in my bathroom. Therefore, each day and each night, I cannot look at myself honestly in the mirror without looking at the Caveman Contract, where I will (hopefully) see all the boxes ticked. Caveman art may not be the sexiest addition to my bathroom decor, but for forty days I must hold myself accountable, and this is the most effective way I can achieve that.

> *Being accountable is about owning my Plan and my body. The battle is largely psychological because I am changing my mentality so that I can own my health. It is my body, my mind, and I am going to stop abusing them both and make a positive change in my lifestyle.*

7

20 Caveman Questions with Annie

I am getting nervous as Day 1 approaches, but I'm equally excited as well. I was hoping a lunch with Annie could calm my nerves a bit.

At this stage, lunch with Annie kind of sucked because knowing that my cheeky eating days are soon to be over, I just want to pig out on pizza and fries. But I wouldn't do that in front of Annie now, would I? Instead, I had to gain some control and look for the chicken burger or equally healthy menu option. I chalked up this lunch as *practice*.

Anyway, I'd warned Annie that I was coming to lunch with questions, so here's how it all panned out:

M: Hello Annie. I like that top you are wearing. Very nice. Every issue of Playboy has a '20 Questions With…' section, so let's play the questions game, okay?
A: *Hi Mike, thanks for the compliment. I'm impressed that you actually read the articles.*

M: Ha ha, good one. So how are you doing today?
A: *Was that question number one?*

M: Nope. Wow you're straight to business today.
A: *Well, I'm here to help you get fit and healthy. Fun begins when that mission is accomplished.*

M: Well, okay then Ms Cheeky Trainer, this is my first question. Physically I am not where I want to be. Based on what you know about my lifestyle, my diet and my workouts leading up to this point, where have I gone wrong?

A: *Well, easy question to ask, but it's a tough one to answer, Mike. Your goal is fitness AND health, and by looking at your past eating, drinking and workout patterns, you've pretty much missed the mark in all areas. We will have to change all three of those elements in your daily life. So, we will need to take a deep breath and move on and start looking to the next forty days. We've designed a Caveman Eating and Workout Plan that I guarantee will overhaul your body and change you, emotionally, for the better.*

M: I'm about to turn 35 years old though. Is it too late?

A: *It's never too late, but at 35 years old, you are like many and most 20 to 50 year olds who haven't been watching what they're eating and who have been drinking too much.*

M: Okay cool. I'm happy to hear that. You know my goal is simple - I want to look good in jeans! I don't need to look like Mr Schwarzenegger. I want to eat better, drink less, sleep better and have better workouts so that I'm happy in my jeans and a t-shirt, and so that I'm not self-conscious on the beach in my Speedos!

A: *Oh my. You wear Speedos?*

M: Actually, no. That was a joke – a bad one at that. Please continue.

A: *Okay, well now that you have a general goal, you just need to follow the Plan until you reach that goal. Your goal is simple, realistic and personal. Just do me a favour and include '100 per cent dedication to sticking to the Caveman Contract' into your goals, and I know you will be very happy with your look at the beach as well as in your jeans and t-shirt at the end of the forty days.*

M: I can do that. What about adopting a BMI goal or other lifestyle measurements out there – are these any good?

A: *An alcoholic who is within the healthy BMI range isn't really that healthy, is he? Also, bodybuilders are considered overweight according to the BMI because it doesn't take into consideration the weight of muscle. So the BMI* *is really just a general guide. Numbers are just numbers – you have told me yourself that you're not chasing biceps that are X centimetres in size, or that you want to weigh X kilograms at the end of the forty days. You are simply trying to get your life back, and I think that by the end of forty days we'll be able to properly assess your progress by some objective means, rather than by using some random number.*

M: I'm afraid I'll get off-track and lose focus. What happens if I do?

A: *Then we sit you down and beat you. Just kidding. We focus on your goals and why you are doing this and the benefits you'll get out of it once you do have your life back on track. Losing your way is normal, but if you stay focused you won't fall off the rails. Stumbling is all part of the process. The key to success is that when you do, you return to the path refocused and ready to work even harder to achieve your goal.*

M: Okay. You have brought up 'change' quite a bit. My problem is: I want to change, but I'm not sure I can. Can you help?

A: *We are constantly changing, so it is not something to fear or worry about. The question is, are we changing for the better or worse? Our goal should always be to achieve constant and never-ending improvement. You can achieve any realistic goal if you genuinely want it and can keep your eye on the final outcome.*

M: That all makes sense, Annie. And in the end, I need to look myself in the mirror and realise that this is my life, and I either get off my arse and make the change, or stay chubby and unhealthy forever. Continuing on, if I follow our City Caveman Plan, what results can I expect?

A: *How does this sound? Better sleep, more energy, better sex, better ability to concentrate, better skin, better times on the toilet, less pressure on your heart, knees, ankles and joints, lower chance of adult diabetes – I could go on and on…*

M: Wow, I'll follow the Caveman rainbow if the pot of gold includes all of that! I want all of that. Is forty days really enough time?

A: *Yes, forty days is enough time for you to start seeing positive changes and develop healthy habits you can keep for life.*

M: Okay. Here's a tough one. I'm carrying at least a good 12 kilograms of chub on my body that I need to lose. 12 kilograms on my frame, or 50 kilograms on another guy/gal – do we have the same battle?

A: *You have the same battle, but yours will be shorter than someone who has to lose 50 kilograms. Essentially, both of you will have to get moving, adopt a new lifestyle and put your health and fitness at the forefront of your mind in order to become healthy again.*

M: You saw my daily eating chart. What is the worst thing about my eating habits?

A: *Well, you tell me by answering this question: what do you normally eat for breakfast?*

M: I don't.

A: *And there is your answer. Breakfast is so important to eat because it gets your metabolism started for the day. Of course, I don't mean eating fried bacon and eggs and having three coffees. I mean having a healthy, nutritious start to your day.*

M: Okay, I get it – breakfast! I promise to change that. Okay, what else?

A: *Your eating is too erratic. Sometimes you eat healthy and sometimes you eat like a pig. You need to eat a low fat diet on a consistent basis to be healthy and lose body fat.*

M: I'm with you. My eating patterns are crap. Vitamin shops are everywhere selling 'bulk up' powders, crazy snake oil and who knows what. Should I be using any of this?

A: *Well, if you educate yourself on what your body needs and what is actually in those 'snake oils', you might find that some may be beneficial in addition to a healthy diet. But, as we are developing a City Caveman Plan for you, fresh, healthy food, along with water and freshly squeezed juice, are ideal, nutritious, tasty ways to stay hydrated and absorb the nutrients your body needs.*

M: What about a low-carb diet or some kind of diet that makes those nightly news shows or women's magazines?

A: *I personally don't think carbs are bad; it's more about the type and quantity that you need to be careful with. Wholemeal options are best. That period where carbs were branded as near poison was just a fad that became blown out of proportion. The bottom line is that diets don't work, so don't bother with any of them.*

M: You and I have spoken about this Cavemen Eating Plan at length. Do you think eating fresh, healthy foods without chemicals (but that aren't necessarily organic) has the makings of being a fad?

A: *Not at all. It's tasty, healthy and realistic. Basic eating can still be fun and tasty, it just takes a little more imagination at times. If your goal is improving your life and fitness, there is only one way to eat – fresh and healthy.*

M: You know I love food. I really have no method in my food selection process other than 'That sounds bloody tasty, so I'll have it.' How do I change this thought process?

A: *You have to start seeing food as fuel rather than food as comfort; and that includes liquids as well. You do have a very high and unhealthy alcohol consumption, which has rewarded you with that beer belly. Let's change your fatty food and beer consumption to lean foods with fresh juice or water, and I assure you, you will start seeing enormous results.*

M: But why does alcohol hurt fitness so much?

A: *Alcohol is a toxin; it's high in empty calories (i.e., calories that provide no nutritional value) and it slows your metabolism. And on top of that, the day after your bender will leave you with a hangover which will have you feeling lethargic all day long while your body tries to rid itself of all those toxins you've consumed.*

M: A bit gross, but to be very blunt and honest, my time on the toilet is best described as hot, wet and fast. Will this change under the City Caveman Plan?

A: *Yes. It will become a calm and solid experience once your health is restored. And another thought for you: if it hurts coming out now, imagine what it is doing to your intestines while it's making its way through your body. Know what I mean?*

M: Definitely. What about snacks? I find it hard to go without something during the day, and how do I turn that cheeky night time snack into something a bit healthier?

A: *Try eating healthy snacks like fruit, dried fruit, rice crackers or carrot and celery sticks.*

M: Would you prescribe the same workout routine for women as well?

A: *Yes. Male or female, the City Caveman Workout Plan we have designed will not cause you to bulk up but, rather, firm up and slim down. Male or female, young or old, this workout is a balance of weights and cardio training which suits everyone. Couple this with the healthy diet of low-fat fresh foods and you've got a very simple but effective recipe for success.*

M: There are so many cardiovascular workout options, from running, to cycling, to swimming and so on. What do you recommend?

A: *I recommend all of the above and anything else that gets your heart rate up. Studies show that running burns more fat than most exercises, and in Australia we have plenty of land to run on, and plenty of gyms in which to hit the treadmill. I would recommend running for you, but that's because you are used to it. Definitely, pick an activity that you enjoy and one that your lower body joints can handle.*

M: I'm semi-allergic to weights. I despise going to that section of the gym. Do you have any tips to ease my pain?

A: *This is a challenge for most people who are new to the gym. Just know that your insecurities about going to that part of the gym will decrease as your habits move from bad to good and as your body image improves. Yes, it's a challenge, but it's one that you'll simply have to overcome and you will find it less and less of a concern as you progress through the Plan and start seeing results.*

M: What do most people do improperly during their workouts?

A: *Socialise too much! Think of your health as important business; nobody likes to waste time socialising when something important is staring them in the face. Also, too many people use poor technique while performing their workouts. Pulling a muscle or hurting your back while doing something improperly can cost you your health for days, weeks, months or even years.*

M: Okay, is there anything that you'd like to address?

A: *Three things to take away for you Mike, and it will guarantee success and health: commit, take ownership and stay focused. Got it?*

M: Yes, I fully understand. Thanks for answering my questions. I'm still nervous but equally excited. Do you want to grab a beer now?

A: *That was more than twenty questions chubby boy. No beer for you. If you're nervous and you're excited, at least I know you've got some energy in there. Lace up those Nikes – we're going for a run!*

8

City Caveman Workout Plan

Day 1: Shoulders, Biceps and Triceps

1 **Warm up:** 3 minutes of jumping rope or 3 minutes on the rowing machine.

2 **20 minutes of cardiovascular activity**: Running, cycling, walking or rowing, etc. It's your choice.

Shoulders

3 Barbell Upright Row *(3 sets of 12 repetitions)*

Holding the bar at shoulder's width apart, pull bar upward to neck level. Lower, then repeat.

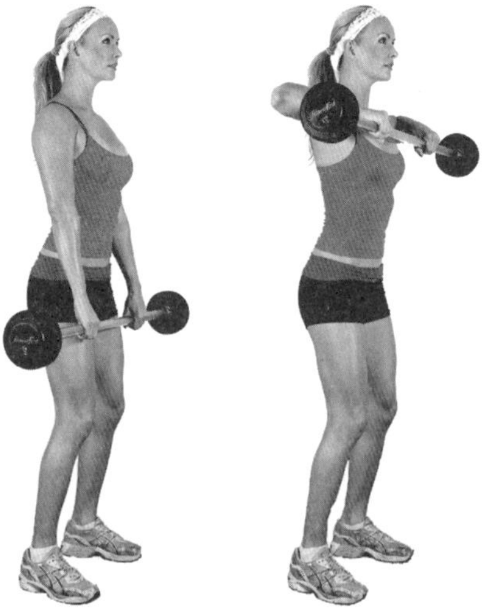

4 Dumbbell Front & Side Raise *(3 sets of 12 repetitions)*

With knees slightly bent, hold dumbbells and raise out in front to shoulder level. Then, extend arms outward to the side and lower.

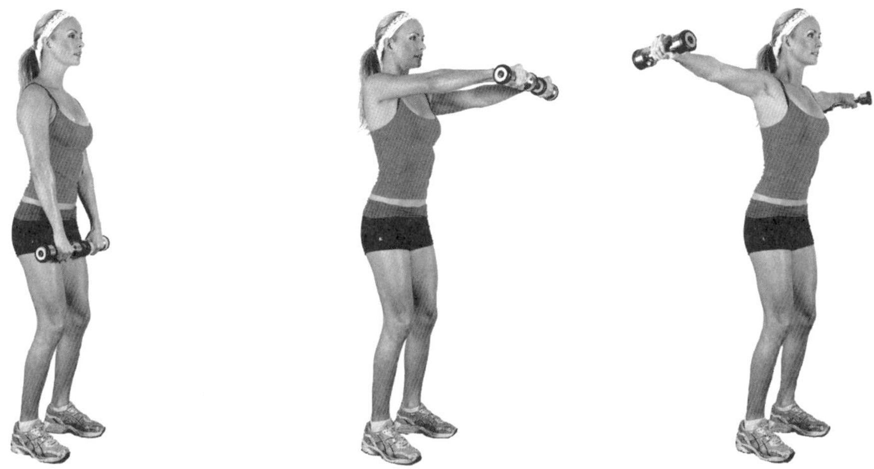

5 Dumbbell Shoulder Press *(3 sets of 12 repetitions)*

Elbows should be positioned below the wrist, and position dumbbells to each side of shoulders. Push dumbbells until arms are extended overhead. Lower, then repeat.

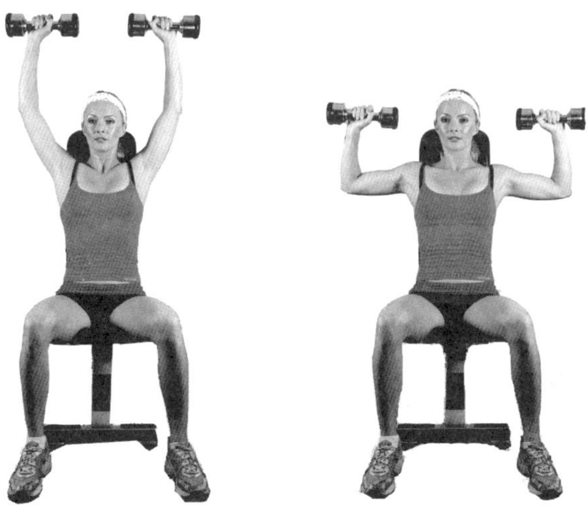

Biceps

6 Barbell Curl *(3 sets of 12 repetitions)*

With an underhand grip, grab bar at shoulder's width, and raise until forearms face shoulder. Lower, then repeat.

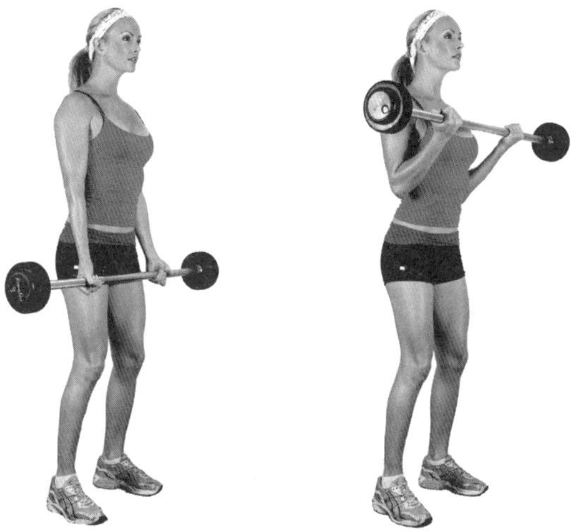

7 Dumbbell Hammer Curl *(3 sets of 12 repetitions)*

With dumbbells on each side, palms facing inward, raise one dumbbell until thumb faces shoulder. Alternate with other arm.

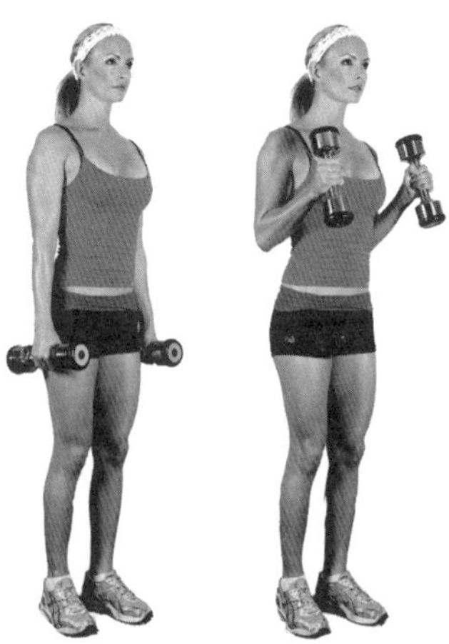

8 Barbell (or machine) Preacher Curl *(3 sets of 12 repetitions)*

With arms on back of pad, grab curl bar with underhand grip, and raise until forearms face shoulder. Lower, then repeat.

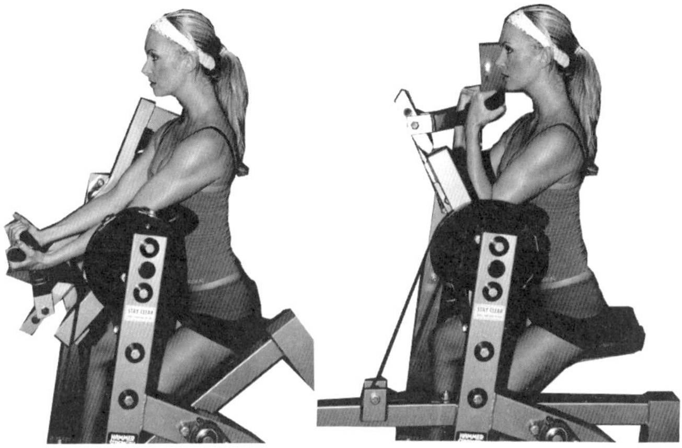

Triceps

9 Tricep Barbell Extension *(3 sets of 12 repetitions)*

Lie on bench, with arms fully extended at the top. Lower barbell to forehead while keeping elbows stationary. Raise to top, then repeat.

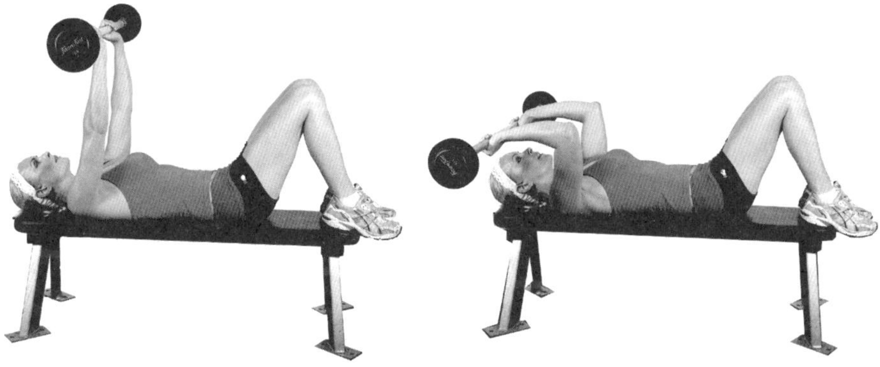

10 Tricep Pull Down *(3 sets of 12 repetitions)*

With knees slightly bent, extend arms downward while keeping elbows close to side. Raise, then repeat.

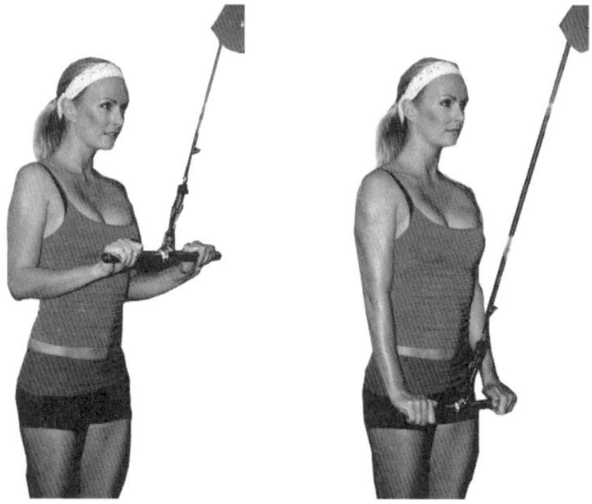

Stretch (5 minutes)

Days 2, 4 & 6: Cardio

1 **Warm up:** 3 minutes of jumping rope or 3 minutes on rowing machine.

2 **40 minutes of cardiovascular activity**: Running, cycling, walking or rowing, etc. It's your choice.

3 **Abdominal Exercises (*10 repetitions, increasing by 2 each week. And remember: squeeze those abs!!!*)**

   a *Reverse Curl* – Elevate knees and align lower legs parallel to the ground. Contracting lower abs, raise hips off the floor, and bring thighs towards chest. Lower, then repeat.

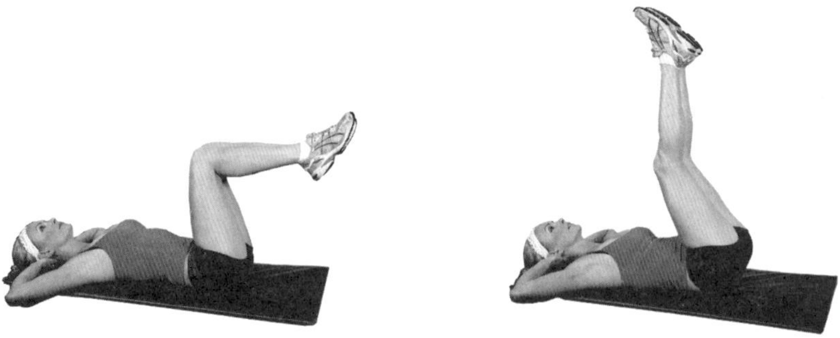

b *Overhead Crunch* – Place hands overhead and interlock grip, and contract abdominal muscles (avoid using neck muscles) to lift body to an angle of 40 degrees. Lower, then repeat.

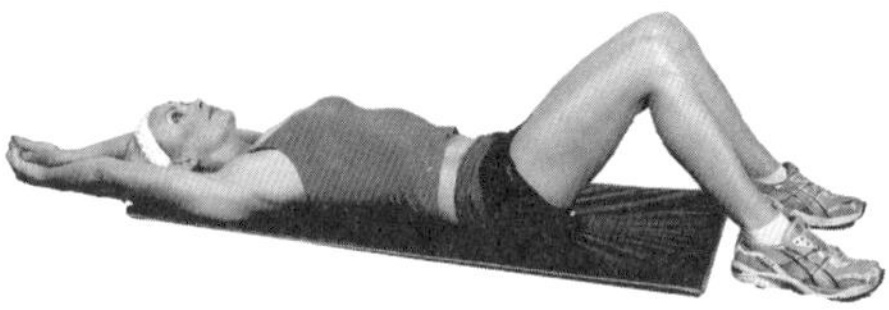
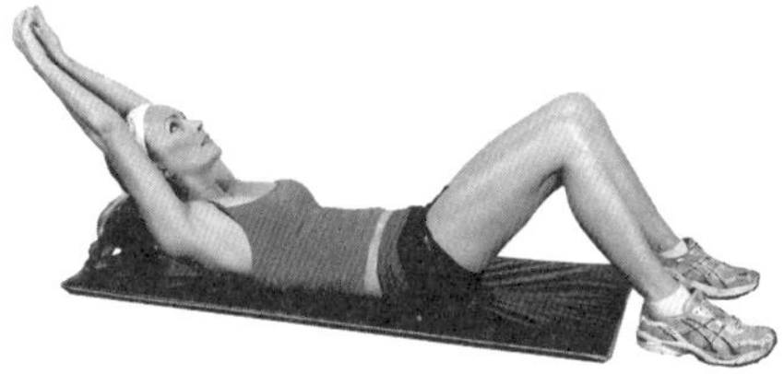

c *Side Crunch* – Starting at the waist, turn legs completely to one side, and crunch straight up. Contract abdominals (obliques), and do not pull on neck. Lower, then repeat. Perform reps, then switch sides.

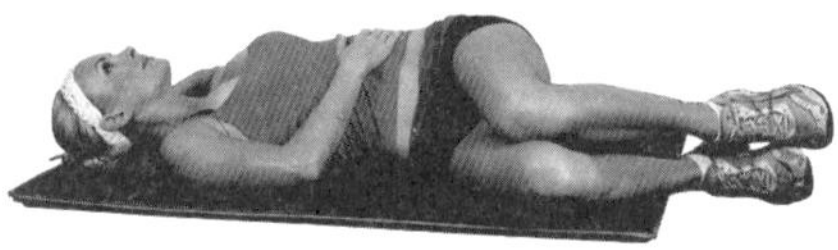
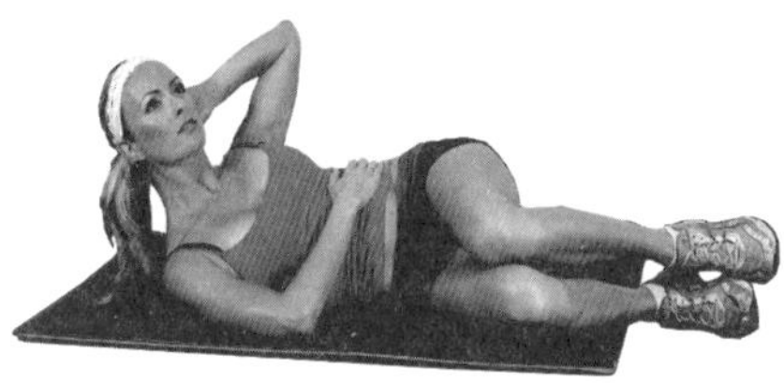

d *Elbow-Knee Crunch* – Bend right leg up and rest right foot on left knee. Contracting abdominals into a sideways crunch, touch left elbow to right knee. Lower, then repeat. Perform reps, then switch sides.

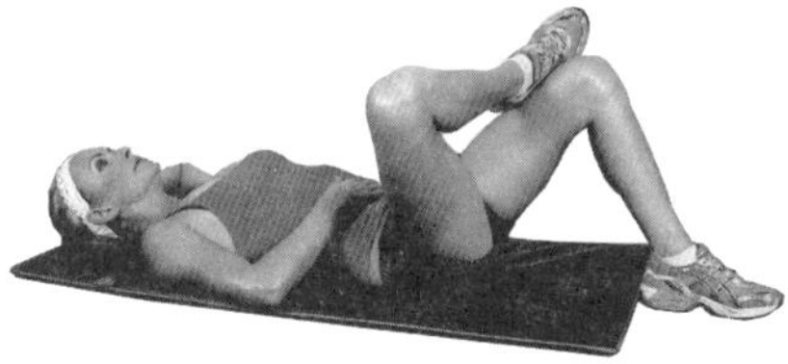
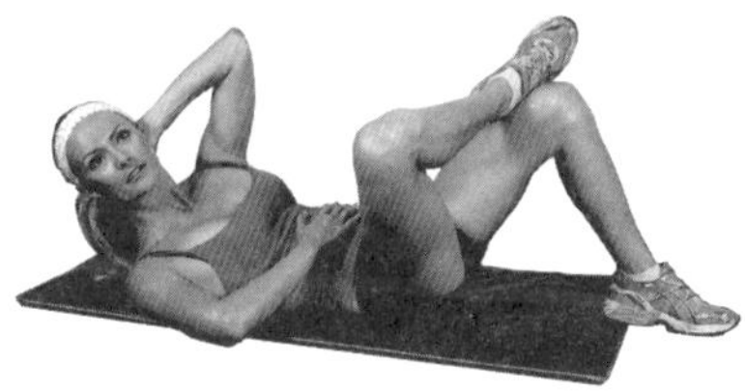

e *Standard Crunch* – Lie face-up with knees bent, feet flat on ground and elbows on the floor. Contract abdominals as if to press navel toward spine, and raise head, neck and shoulderblades off ground as a single unit. Lower, then repeat.

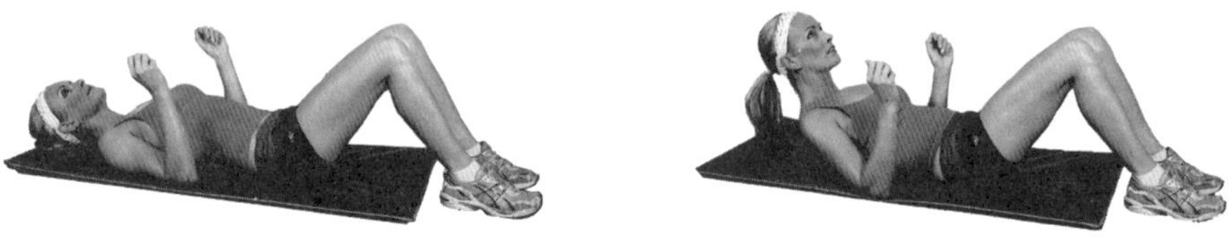

Stretch (5 minutes)

Day 3: Legs

1 **Warm up:** 3 minutes of skipping rope or 3 minutes on rowing machine.

2 **20 minutes of cardiovascular activity**: Running, cycling, walking or rowing, etc. It's your choice.

3 **Squats *(3 sets of 12 repetitions)***
Stand with dumbbells at sides and feet shoulder-width apart. Descend to the squat position while knees are pointing in the same direction as feet. Return to starting position, then repeat.

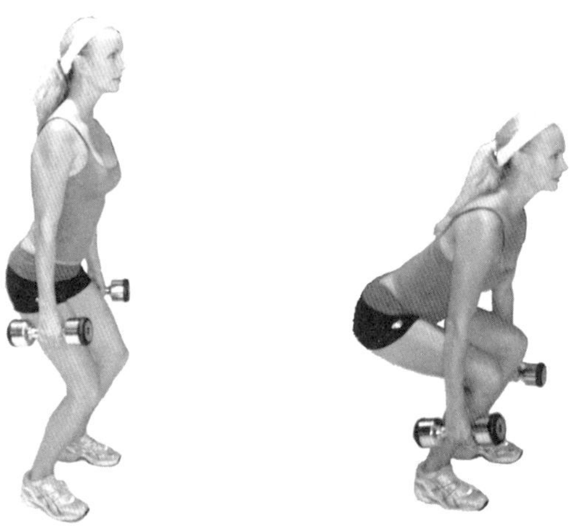

4 Leg Extension ***(3 sets of 12 repetitions)***

Sit and extend knees until legs are straight. Lower, then repeat.

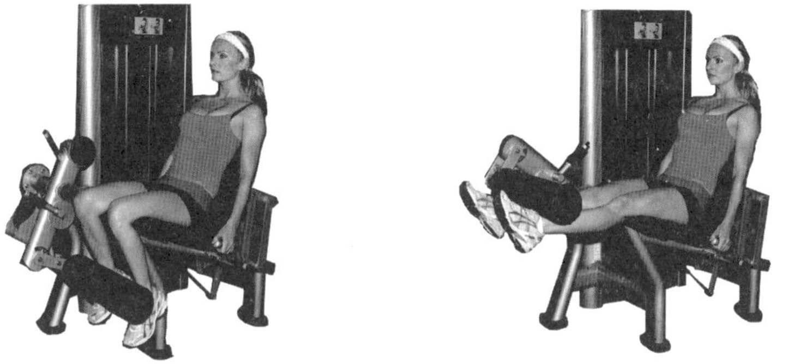

5 Butt Kickback ***(2 sets of 20 with each leg)***

On hands and knees with back parallel to the ground, thrust feet backward and upward. Lower to beginning position, then repeat.

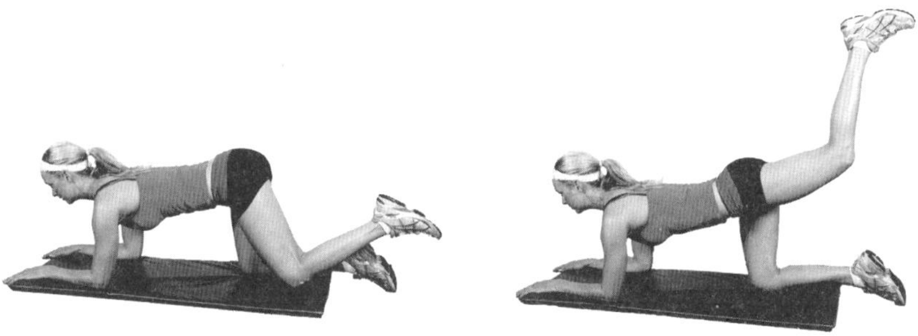

6 Leg Curl ***(3 sets of 12 repetitions)***

Lying face down and grasping handles, raise pad at lower calf until it hits back of thighs. Lower until knees are straight, then repeat.

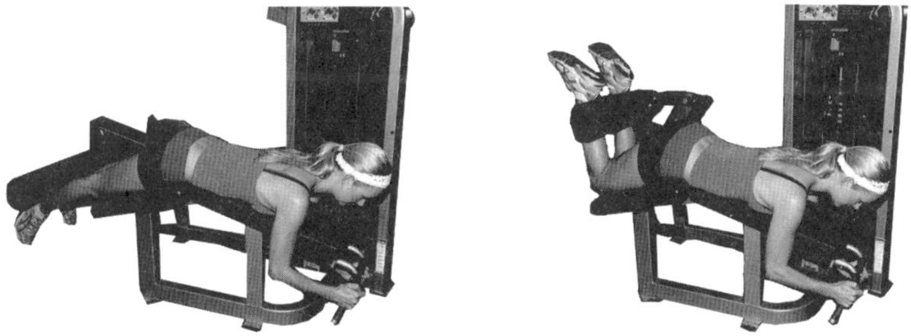

7 Dumbbell Lunge *(3 sets of 12 with each leg)*

Holding dumbbells with relaxed shoulders, lunge downward with first leg until knee is at 90 degrees. Raise until just before knees are locked, then repeat.

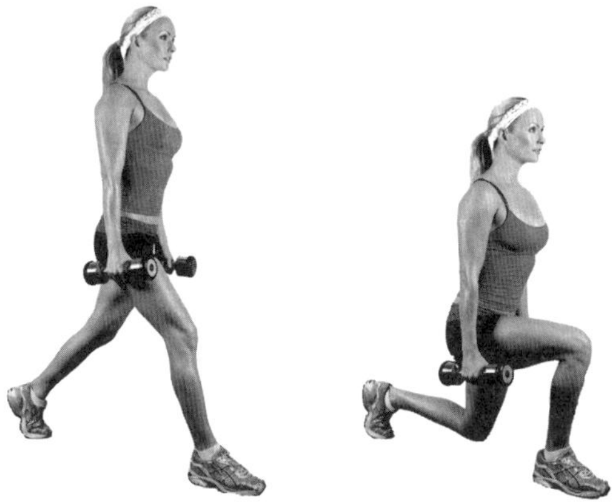

Stretch (5 minutes)

Day 5: Chest and Back

1 Warm up: 3 minutes of jumping rope or 3 minutes on rowing machine.

2 20 minutes of cardiovascular activity: Running, cycling, walking or rowing, etc. It's your choice.

Chest

3 Bench Press *(3 sets of 12 repetitions)*

Lying down on a bench, lift barbell from rack using a wide grip. Lower weight to upper chest but avoid hitting chest. Lift until arms are extended, then repeat. For safety, please use a spotter or, if no one is available, use a machine.

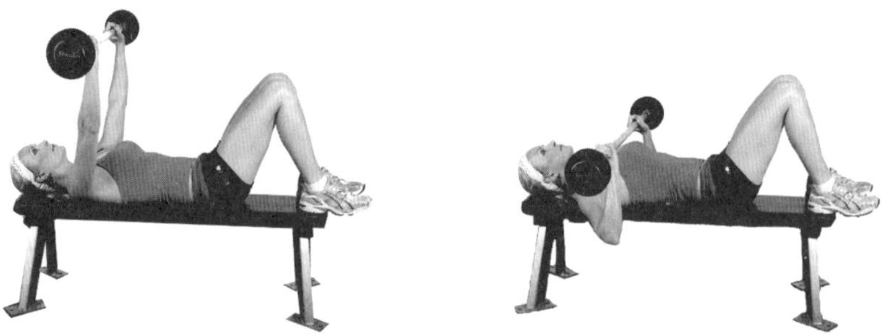

4 Incline Bench Press *(3 sets of 12 repetitions)*

Lying down on an inclined bench, lift barbell from rack using a wide grip. Lower weight to upper chest but avoid hitting chest. Lift until arms are extended, then repeat. For safety, please use a spotter or, if no one is available, use a machine.

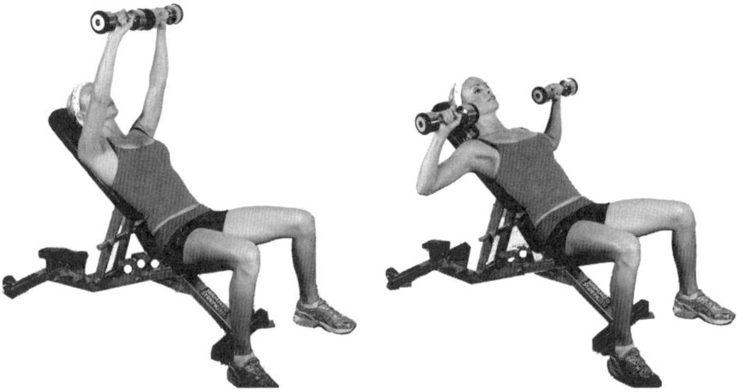

5 Fly Bench *(3 sets of 12 repetitions)*

Raise dumbbells above chest with arms fixed in a slightly bent position. Lower dumbbells to sides with elbows staying fixed. Bring dumbbells together until dumbbells are nearly together, then repeat. For safety, please use a spotter or, if no one is available, use a machine.

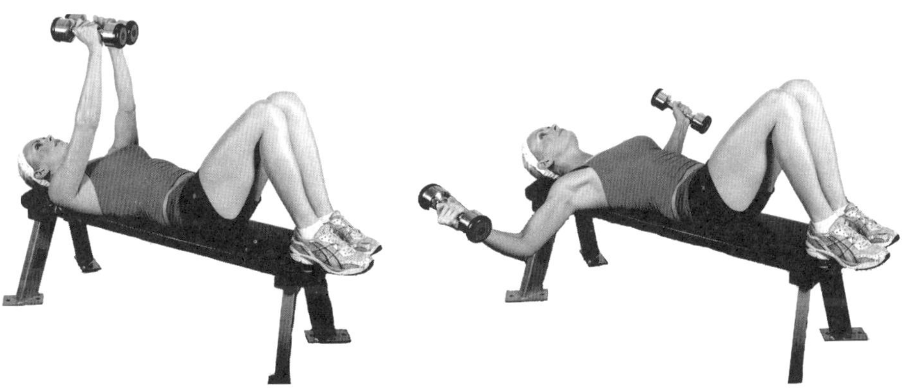

Back

6 Seated Row *(3 sets of 12 repetitions)*

Sit on seat and pull bars back until shoulders are pulled back. Pull weights back until elbows are behind back, and return to original position, then repeat.

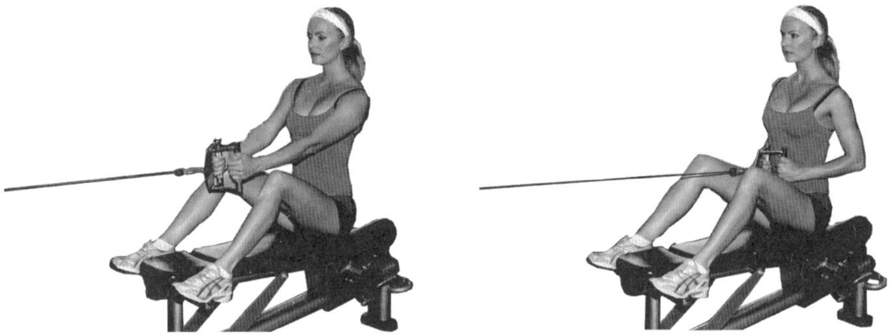

Day 7: Rest and Recovery

Enjoy the day off. Mentally and physically your body needs a rest day.

9

City Caveman Recipes

I am now writing from the post-forty days period because it is appropriate to share some recipes that helped me achieve success.

Keep in mind that these recipes are merely a suggestion, because the City Caveman Plan is exactly that – a plan. And everyone is different, so feel free to try some of the recipes that I used, even if only to see that healthy, tasty food that is full of flavour *does* exist. But you can also use these recipes to create your own delightful treats. And, by doing your own shopping, you will learn and educate yourself about what's good (and bad) for your body, just like I did.

Rita Cozzi is an author, trainer, organic food advocate and naturopathic practitioner, with qualifications in Health Science, Naturopathy and Nursing. Her passionate, fun and interactive method of communicating has led her to explore the power of what we put in our mouths and why this does influence our outcomes. Rita has given over 1,000 presentations, workshops and training programs on health and lifestyle education to health professionals, company executives and community groups nationally and internationally, and this experience uniquely underpins her team-building workshops. As a recognised Clinical Nutrition Advisor, Rita has led effective product design and implementation for Blackmores and designed and conducted technical seminars and briefings for health professionals to help continuously improve outcomes.

I sought Rita's professional advice, to ensure our recipes were worthy of a Caveman Stamp of Approval, and to provide insight as to how and why these recipes are good for our minds, bodies and overall health.

Breakfast

I knew that going from habitually eating no breakfast to eating breakfast every day would be quite a significant lifestyle change for me, but within my forty days, I quickly found that a great, healthy and tasty way to start the day was to make a morning smoothie. If I knew I was in for a busy week, I could cut the fruit up on Sunday, and I found I could make a smoothie in two minutes, drink it, then head straight out the door. It wasn't nearly as time consuming as I'd expected it would be!

Here are a few super tasty, low fat options that worked for me:

Citrus Smoothie

1 cup orange juice
1 cup pineapple juice
1 banana
1 cup ice

Banana Berry Smoothie

1 banana
1/4 cup berries
1 1/2 cups skim milk
1 pear

Berry Berry Smoothie

1 cup frozen forest berries
3/4 cup pineapple juice
1 cup of skim milk

Kiwi-ana Smoothie

1 1/2 cups skim milk
1 banana
1 pear
1 kiwi

Berri-ango Smoothie

1/2 cup frozen forest berries
1/2 cup fresh or frozen mango
1 cup orange juice

On the mornings where I had a bit more time, I'd enjoy an egg-white omelette (one whole egg and three egg whites) with some prawns, garlic, mushrooms and ground black pepper. Or, if I had an itching for a little bread, I prepared organic, seeded brown bread with some fresh avocado and ground black pepper along with a banana and freshly squeezed orange juice. It was all delicious and it made me feel so much better in the mornings!

Rita says: I consult too many clients who all say the same thing – 'I don't have time for breakfast.' Huge mistake. No meal should be missed, and when taking on an appropriate fitness plan, you will need all the energy you can get from a balanced nutrition program; a healthy breakfast is the only way to start one's day.

Unfortunately we are not getting enough fruit in our diets in today's culture, and one of the most nutritious ways of starting the day is with a healthy fruit smoothie. Why eat fruit? Because it is a great source of dietary fibre, and those who consume it have a reduced risk of chronic disease. Each fruit has its own unique properties, and the natural sugars contained in fruit are a healthier source of sugar compared to the refined sugars which are devoid of natural vitamins and minerals. Remember two to three pieces of fruit per day is a great guide to ensure you get lots of nutrients.

In addition to the City Caveman smoothies, some individuals might find that additional morning protein helps maintain blood sugar levels and mental energy up to lunchtime. Some additions to the City Caveman smoothies can be an egg (blended), almonds (or almond milk), or seed mix – all of which provide high quality sources of protein. Beware of 'healthy' smoothies at the local shopping mall, as many of them include added syrup and/or ice cream, which are not a very healthy start to one's day, nor is it actually part of your City Caveman Eating Plan.

Remember, fruit is a great source of fibre, vitamins, minerals and antioxidants. Eating fruits in season ensures optimum nutritional value, which will help maintain healthy gums, eyes, skin, lungs and immune function and, of course, give us all the fibre that comes with natural fruit.

For this reason, unless the juice is freshly made and some of the pulp is retained, I recommend that fresh fruit juices be squeezed in preference to the packaged juices, which are often adulterated with added sugar – sometimes more than a can of soft drink! None of us needs this extra sugar, and this is actually where some diets fall over; the sugar equates to extra calories, which is then stored as excess fat.

Water

Whenever I chat about the City Caveman Plan, water seems to be the one thing where people proclaim, 'Oh wow, consuming two litres of water will be a tough one.'

What the hell?

It's just water, so why is it so hard for people to swallow the concept?

I think in today's culture, we fill up on coffee in the morning, Coke and sugar-laced juices during the day, and night time is about a beer or wine, or two. We've fallen out of the habit when it comes to drinking the right amount of water each day.

Well, it's time for a change, and so here are my tips on consuming an appropriate amount of water:

a Consume a 600ml bottle of water before you leave the house in the morning.
b Consume at least a 600ml bottle of water during your workouts. You must keep yourself hydrated! Your mind and your muscles will thank you for it.
c And that leaves the entire rest of the day to have 800ml of water. See? It's not so tough after all, is it?

If you need some flavour, try squeezing some lemon into your water. Also, I once had cucumber slices put in my water at a nice restaurant, and I was sold – I love it. I found quickly during my City Caveman Plan that cold water was hard to consume in mass unless I was working out, so I switched to room temperature water during the day, and it seems to go down so much more easily. But everyone's different.

Rita says: The human body is made up of around 65 per cent water, and two-thirds of the earth is made up water as well. It sounds simple, doesn't it? Living things need water in order to survive and stay healthy. Among its accolades, water keeps us hydrated, decreases the pain that dehydration can cause in our muscles and joints, regulates our body temperature and also transports oxygen to our cells. Admittedly, I sometimes struggle to consume two litres of water every day too, but there is no question that we must manage at least one to one-and-a-half litres of water a day while keeping in mind the good tips Mike has outlined. Fruit, salad and other foods contain water, so other healthy food can also assist in replacing fluids lost during a full day.

Lunch

Sometimes lunch can be a tough one. It would be great to make something the night before to have a yummy treat the following day, but who really has the time, right? And, if you're an 8am to 5pm worker, it's difficult to find the kitchen facilities it takes to get super creative in the kitchen.

So, if you don't have leftovers from the night before to enjoy, then the easy sandwich or quick salad should become your best lunch friend. I'm only asking that you put down the prime-rib-steak knife and fork for that boozy business lunch and give the fast food burgers a miss for forty days! Trust me, you're going to love the results if you do. Plus, instead of having a huge lunch and diving into a food coma afterwards because you are so full, you're going to find yourself with so much more energy throughout your day.

A favourite sandwich of mine is made from organic, seeded brown bread (low fat wraps or rice cakes are also a good substitute), which I would fill with sliced veggies; anything from cucumber, avocado, tomatoes, onion, spinach leaves, rocket leaves. And add to them, chicken breast or lean beef, topped with seeded mustard, and there you have it! A healthy lunch that will keep you full and tantalise your tastebuds.

I also found that keeping a fat-free dressing in the fridge was a great substitute for mayo or that thick dose of butter that I might normally put on a sandwich. Sure, I missed that slice of cheese, but in order to keep a sandwich low in fat, it's best to keep it cheese-free. Along with a piece of fruit and big glass of water, I was always full and happy after a healthy sandwich like this.

Also, I found that salads with any choice of lettuce leaf could be made in a healthy, tasty manner, be it for lunch or dinner. And by adding salmon, lean meat or chicken breast, I was able to stick to the 10 grams of fat limitation with ease. And salad dressing didn't just have to just be a splash of lemon juice; sometimes I experimented. Here are a few fat-free, healthy salad dressings to spice up your meal:

Cucumber Dill

1 small fat free yoghurt
Chopped cucumbers
1 bunch green onions
2 tsp dill
Garlic to taste
Squeeze of lemon

Mango Orange

1 medium mango in chunks
1/2 cup fresh orange juice
1 clove garlic, crushed
1 teaspoon soy sauce
1/4 teaspoon curry powder

Vinegar Dijon

1 clove garlic, minced
3 tbsp red wine vinegar
1-2 tbsp dijon mustard
1 tsp salt
1/2 tsp ground pepper

Basil Vinaigrette

1/4 cup balsamic vinegar
1/4 tsp dried basil
1/4 tsp dried oregano
Splash of lemon juice

Honey-Mustard

Big spoon of mustard
Big spoon of honey
Splash of balsamic

Of course, during my forty days, I didn't get a chance to make lunch or consume healthy leftovers every day so I did have to learn how to deal with the temptations of all those cheeky treats and non-Caveman foods when I needed to buy my lunch out and about.

I learned that there are plenty of healthy options if you look in the right places. Yes, it can be a real battle to say 'no' when your co-workers are having the red curry with duck, but we've all signed up for a different plan over forty days. Be it a healthy sandwich on brown bread, salmon and avocado sushi rolls, rice paper rolls with prawn, or a fresh salad with low fat dressing, there are healthy options at restaurants and food courts that will allow you to stay true to the City Caveman Plan. You just have to remember to choose them!

Rita says: Mike's dressings are a great option to enhance flavour for salads, and I strongly urge you to use avocado, as well as tuna in spring water, hummus or tahini on your salad or wrap, to add variety and broaden the nutritional spectrum. Low fat cheese such as ricotta or cottage may also provide desirable options for salads or wraps. Other options could include a small helping of chick peas, which can be added to any salad for more sustenance when chicken, turkey or tuna are not available or desirable.

I also find that pre-making a Sunday, ready-to-go serve of delicious soup such as minestrone, pumpkin or lentil is ideal to have handy throughout the working week and this would fit well within the City Caveman Plan. Some of my tasty soup recipes are detailed below:

Minestrone Soup	
2 cloves garlic, finely chopped 2 medium onions, finely sliced 1 cup celery, chopped 3 carrots, finely chopped 3 zucchini, finely chopped 3 fresh, ripe tomatoes, diced 3 tbsp tomato paste 4 cups chicken, beef or vegetable stocks 1 cup cooked brown rice 3 cups cooked beans (borlotti or cannellini) 2 tbsp fresh oregano, finely chopped Freshly ground black pepper	*Place onion, garlic and celery in a large saucepan with 2 cups of stock. Simmer for 15 minutes. Add all ingredients to the saucepan except oregano and pepper. Simmer covered for a further 30 to 45 minutes. The soup may be pureed in a blender or left as is, adding fresh pepper and oregano and simmering a further 5 minutes. Serve hot. Serves 4–6.*

Lentil Soup	
2 cloves garlic 2 medium onions 1 bay leaf Freshly ground nutmeg ½ cup parsley, finely chopped 3 cups vegetable stock 3 cups dried brown lentils 1–2 cups water	*Place onion and garlic in large saucepan with 1 cup of stock and simmer for 10 minutes. Add 1 cup of water and remaining vegetable stock and the lentils. Allow to simmer for 20 to 30 minutes and check, as more water may be required (½ to 1 cup depending on uptake of lentils). Taste to check that lentils are soft. If so, add parsley, nutmeg and bay leaf. Simmer for a further 5 minutes and serve hot. Serves 2–3.*

Pumpkin Soup	
2 medium onions, finely sliced 3 medium carrots, scrubbed and finely diced ½ small pumpkin, cleaned and chopped 2 medium sweet potatoes, peeled and finely diced 4 cups defatted chicken, beef or vegetable stock Freshly ground black pepper 1 tsp turmeric 1 tsp coriander Fresh coriander for serving	*Place onions, carrots, sweet potato and pumpkin in 3 cups of the stock in a large stock saucepan and simmer for 30 minutes. Add last cup of stock and more water if desired and cook further 20 minutes. Add pepper, turmeric and coriander and blend. Pour soup back into saucepan and serve hot with a garnish of fresh coriander, if available. Serves 6-8.*

Snacks

Need a snack in the morning or late afternoon? I recommend:

8 Snack Options	
Cut up apple No fat vanilla yoghurt Walnuts	Dried fruit (Found in health food stores)
No fat yoghurt	Dry nuts
Carrots and celery	Sultanas
Rice crackers	Popcorn

It was difficult to give up the chocolate, potato chips and fast food snack packs. But as the days went by and I continued to win my daily battles, my tastebuds changed, and healthy snacks were actually a nice change from the greasy, fatty treats of the past.

Dinner

With just a little extra thought, I was able to create some damn good City Caveman dinners. Remember, this Plan is not a diet or a program about restrictions. It is about refocusing and getting back on track with tasty, healthy and fresh eating, and I was able to do this without ever feeling hungry at the end of a night. Sure, some days I wanted fish and chips with more than a dash of salt, but I battled wisely by choosing fresh salmon on a bed of veggies instead. And instead of going to bed with a gut full of naughty meals, I went to bed every night feeling fresh, full and healthier than the day before.

Here are some of the dinner recipes I used:

Caveman Chicken Chilli	
250g chicken breast (skinless) ½ cup onions, chopped 4 vine-ripened tomatoes ½ cup red capsicum, chopped (Chop up any other veggies you like: mushrooms, cucumber...the options are endless.) ½ can dark red kidney beans ½ jar organic spaghetti sauce 2 cloves garlic Pinch of cumin Pinch or two of black pepper 1 tbsp chilli powder	*In a wok, cook the garlic, onion and chicken. Then add everything else and cook for 20 to 30 minutes on high until you obtain the consistency you prefer. Chilli in a wok? I know it sounds crazy, but it's just so easy to throw it all in! Normally, of course, chilli is filled with cheese and sour cream, but I'm stripping all the fat grams out without losing any of the great flavour of chilli. I love this recipe – it fills you up, it's tasty and healthy; it's the ideal City Caveman Plan food. Serves 2–3.*

Rita says: Why chilli? *Vine-ripened tomatoes can help give your skin a healthy glow as they contain the skin-nurturing nutrients, beta carotene and Vitamin E. Tomatoes are also rich in lycopene, which protects against a range of cancers. Chilli is warming and stimulates the blood, lymph nodes and circulation but may also induce sweating in some depending on the heat of the chilli, so be careful!*

Growing up in Dad's restaurant, I was always a meat-only eater. Fish? No chance. I couldn't stomach any of it. I must have been around 21 years old when I first dared to try seafood, such as prawns, lobster and fish. I became a convert; I loved the taste of fish. Unfortunately though, my love for aquamarine life has made me try one too many unhealthy fish-and-chip shops throughout Australia! But, for a great, quick and easy salmon, the way nature intended, try this recipe. You can also use chicken or tuna steaks to add variety:

Grilled Salmon with Asian Veggies
Put some soy sauce, black pepper and crushed garlic into a bowl and mix well. Add the salmon and rub in the soy and garlic marinade. Let the salmon sit for 10 minutes (you can let it sit in the fridge all day if you'd like the marinade to soak in for even more taste), and then cook on a healthy grill until medium/medium rare. Serve on 3 handfuls of green, Asian veggies.
Note: Salmon is known as the best brain food, so you'll be a smarter Caveman when you wake up in the morning!

Rita says: Why salmon? *Protein! Salmon also contains omega-3 fatty acids that are thought to protect against heart disease, inflammation, certain types of cancer, diabetes and Alzheimer's disease. Omega-3 fatty acids are critical for proper brain development and neurological function in developing babies, too. And on a lighter note, we should eat salmon because Australia has some of the freshest, tastiest salmon in the world! Salmon is accompanied nicely by a salad or roast veggies done very quickly in a very hot oven, such as carrots, beetroot, red onions and sweet potato. Clean and cut one portion of vegetables into small pieces and drizzle them with a little balsamic vinegar to create another simple and healthy way to compliment a portion of salmon.*

Wholemeal Pasta with Veggies	
4 handfuls wholemeal organic penne pasta 1½ cups organic tomato pasta sauce 2 cups chopped veggies: mushrooms, capsicum, onion, cucumber Freshly ground black pepper ½ clove garlic, crushed	*Cook and drain the wholemeal pasta in one pan, and in another pan heat up the pasta sauce and add all the veggies until cooked nicely. When cooked, add in the pasta and stir thoroughly so the sauce covers your healthy pasta, and enjoy!*

This is the perfect example of our Caveman transformation which strips down our food to simplistic terms. Pre-Plan, my pasta order would have been a cream-based, fat-laden number, also known as the 'Italian Heart Attack'. Strip down that egg pasta and creamy sauce and replace it with tomato and spice – saving us approximately 60 grams of fat, and adding all the nutrition from healthy veggies. You can still enjoy your pasta on the City Caveman Plan, you just have to be a little more creative when putting your health first. Of course, feel free to add a few prawns, scallops or a chicken breast if you feel like making it a seafood or chicken night!

Rita says: Why wholemeal? *Whether in your bread or your pasta, wholemeal (also known as wholegrain) is your best choice. It's low in saturated fat and contains omega-3 fatty acids. It is an excellent source of carbohydrates, a significant source of protein and a good source of many minerals, such as iron, copper, phosphorus* *and zinc. Furthermore, a red sauce is always a better choice than a creamy white sauce because the fat content of cream is through the roof and will likely exceed your daily City Caveman fat allowance.*

Chicken Stir Fry	
You can also try this one with prawns or salmon. 1½ cups brown rice 300g chicken breast (skinless) 4 cups chopped veggies: bok choy, mushrooms, cucumber, capsicum, onion Freshly ground black pepper ½ clove garlic, crushed ¼ cup soy sauce 1 tbsp honey 1 tsp cumin	*In a wok or pan, cook the chicken, then add the soy, garlic, honey, cumin and veggies. Cook until veggies soften. In another pot, boil the brown rice (brown rice is firmer and takes a good 20 to 30 minutes to absorb the water). When the rice is cooked, put into a bowl and serve the chicken with the veggies over the top! Serves 2.*

For too many years, I've eaten the second-rate food filled with MSG, sugar and salt that is served at Asian food stalls in malls across America and Sydney. With just a little thought, you can make Asian food that is just as tasty but ten times healthier. A simple stir fry can be packed with nutrition from the veggies and protein from the chicken.

Rita says: Why brown rice? *Not many people are knowledgeable on why white rice is actually white. It actually starts brown, but it is polished to convert it to its white colour. And it is during that polishing process where the important vitamins and minerals and all of the dietary fibre and essential fatty acids are destroyed. So, when it comes to your rice, if you want to go healthy, then go brown. A combination of wild rice is also nutritious and can be a nice extra option for rice lovers.*

Flavouring additives, such as sodium glutamate are ubiquitous in every one of our pre-packaged sauces, including sweet chilli, and sweet and sour and fish sauces used in Asian restaurants and takeaway shops. Glutamate may be added to foods in relatively large amounts as a flavour enhancer (e.g., MSG or food additives numbered 620 to 625). Some people may have allergic reactions to these food additives and, in some individuals, MSG can even trigger or initiate an asthma attack. As part of the City Caveman eating plan, check labels and avoid MSG and other artificial flavourings wherever possible.

Veggie Salad with Grilled Salmon
Easy! Grill the salmon and cut into strips. Cut up a host of veggies, divide spinach into bowl, and make your favourite salad dressing from our earlier list. Combine it all, and enjoy!

Rita says: Why a salad? *It is good to continue highlighting different salad options, because people should understand that salads can be tasty and filling, and that salad dressings do not have to be loaded with fat. For too long we've been ordering fattening Caesar salad or that chicken schnitzel salad with creamy ranch dressing. If you think those are healthy salad options, think again. The creamy dressings add as much fat as any fast food meal of your liking. Replace it with the fat-free cucumber and dill dressing that Mike detailed earlier, and you'll have just as much taste but with a lot less fat.*

And why spinach? *Spinach is fully loaded with antioxidants that help everything from lowering your risk of ovarian or prostate cancer, to helping your eyesight and providing nutrients for your brain. The abundance of iron from spinach was good enough for Popeye, so it's good enough for you, City Cavemen!*

Grilled Tuna with Avocado & Pineapple Salsa	
400g tuna *For the salsa:* 2 vine-ripened tomatoes, diced ½ small white or Spanish onion, diced Fresh coriander, chopped Freshly ground black pepper Chilli flakes ¼ avocado, in chunks Pineapple chunks Crushed garlic	*Add tomatoes and onion to a bowl with the coriander. Stir gently. Add some pepper and chilli flakes to taste and stir again. Then stir pineapple and avocado chunks into your salsa.* *Rub garlic into the tuna, grill the tuna to medium/medium rare. Serve on top of a rocket salad with balsamic and lemon and drizzle your salsa over the top. Yum! Serves 2.*

Rita says: Why tuna? *Tuna is loaded with healthy nutrients, from protein to Vitamin B to the 'good' cholesterol, HDL. Fish, such as tuna, has been proven to lower the risk of stroke and inflammation within the body. Tuna is a good source of omega-3, which has so many benefits, from helping our skin to improving our heart health. Tuna is also ideal because it can be consumed all year around with healthy canned options for lunch, as well as the fresh tuna caught here in Australia.*

And why avocados? *Avocado is actually a fruit, which contains vitamins A, B, C and E, as well as a healthy dose of fibre. Do be careful as avocados are high in calories and fat, but on a good note, it is the good monounsaturated fat. And some fat is necessary in every diet to maintain brain function and hormone balance.*

Cajun Prawn Skewers	
You can also try using chicken or lamb. 16 prawns, de-veined Cajun spice Crushed garlic Lemon 1 cup brown rice 1 vine-ripened tomato, finely diced 1 green capsicum, cut into 3cm squares 1 white onion, cut into 3cm squares 2 vine-ripened tomatoes, cut into cubes Pineapple chunks	*While the brown rice is boiling, mix 3 tablespoons of Cajun spice (taste to see that it's not too salty), one clove of crushed garlic and a nice splash of lemon juice in a bowl and set aside.* *For the skewers, slide on a prawn, then alternate with the other ingredients, such as onion, tomato, prawn, capsicum, pineapple and so on, and be sure to finish each skewer with a prawn. I was able to get 4 prawns per skewer – see how you go! Then, drizzle over your Cajun spices, and cook the skewers on the grill.* *When the rice is cooked, stir in the finely diced tomato. Enjoy your skewers over the healthy brown tomato rice. I love the sweet and spicy flavour that is created with the blend of the Cajun spice and pineapple. Serves 2.*

Rita says: Why prawns? *Again, omega-3! Omega-3 has been proven to reduce the risk of Alzheimer's and cancer. Some people avoid prawns because they are a little higher in cholesterol, but on the beneficial side, they are packed with low-fat protein.*

Spiced Lamb	
500g lean lamb loin ¼ cup lemon juice 1 tsp oregano 1 tsp thyme 1 tsp freshly ground black pepper ½ tsp cumin 1 tsp parsley	*Squeeze lemon juice into a bowl, then add oregano, thyme, black pepper, parsley and a little hint of cumin. Stir nicely and pour over the lamb loin and let settle for 20 minutes or all day if you have time! Grill the lamb to your liking (I usually try for medium). Prepare a fresh salad to have on the side. Make sure it's loaded with tomatoes, onions, capsicum and a healthy honey-mustard dressing. Serves 2.* *Note: I am a big fan of those healthy indoor grills. Not only does the fat and grease roll off, but they cook just about anything in around four minutes, from steak to fish, to veggies. It will certainly make your life easier to have one while on the City Caveman Plan.*

Rita says: Why lamb? *Lamb is high in protein, which is essential for muscle building and maintaining healthy nails, hair and skin. Protein provides energy for the body. The right meat choice can be very healthy, it just takes a little time to understand which cuts of lamb or steak are lower in fat. The most tender cuts are usually the fattiest, which is bad news, but with a little splash of spice, you can have just as tasty a meal with the additional health benefits!*

Lemon Chicken with Vegetables	
500g chicken breast (skinless) 1 cup organic lemon yoghurt 1 clove garlic Freshly ground black pepper 1 tbsp paprika 1 tsp chilli flakes 5 cups Asian green veggies 1 bunch bok choy, chopped Soy sauce	*In a bowl, crush the garlic, then add yoghurt, paprika, pepper and chilli flakes. Stir, then spread evenly over the chicken breast, and grill or bake.* *In a pan, add a splash of soy to taste, and dump in your veggies and bok choy. Once cooked, serve with the chicken breast. Serves 2.* *It took me a little time during my own City Caveman Plan to realise that the frozen section contains a bit more than pizza, ice cream and other cheeky treats. There are actually great assortments of frozen veggies! And the big food companies have quite a few frozen vegetable options that are great when you're in a time crunch, and even frozen organic veggies can be found. They're chopped up, chemical free and there are plenty of varieties to suit your tastes for the day. Don't pass them up.*

Why lemon chicken with Asian veggies?: *Okay, let's give Rita a break with the nutritional spiel for this recipe because, to be honest, this meal was thrown together when I didn't have time to plan or cook much! I just played it by ear, and within 10 minutes, I had a really, really nice meal of lemon chicken with spices and a bed of healthy veggies. It just took a little thought and a bit of imagination, and it confirms that we can create great food, fast!*

Rita says: *What I like most about the City Caveman mentality is the 'less additives and toxins' approach, because these things are hidden in so much of our everyday food. It is up to us to stop and read the labels of the food we consume.*

Mike is right in saying that we can reduce the intake of so much of these toxins simply by going fresh on a daily basis and, where possible, organic so that added layer of toxins – namely the pesticides, insecticides and herbicides – are actually removed from our daily intake. By following a fresh food plan, such as the City

Caveman Plan, you are more likely to see long-term benefits for your wellbeing and, depending on your genetic history, even on the risk of chronic disease and premature ageing.

An eating plan like the City Caveman Plan is a great starting point for us to refocus and think about what we buy and what we eat.

Real food is becoming increasingly rare in our Western, modern, industrial society, and the development of nutrition as a science has been a double-edged sword, because we see not only greater analysis and understanding of what we eat, but also the effect it has on our bodies. As a nation, we have never been fatter or sicker than since the 'science of food' evolved. In essence, although we have become smarter about our food, we have simultaneously become more obese.

Couple our poor nutrition with the fact we drive when we should be walking, we ride lifts when we should be taking the stairs, and the City Caveman Plan becomes even more significant. Many of us are sedentary during our day jobs and, so, we must check our portions to avoid overeating, understand what we're putting into our bodies and also maintain a moderate regime of exercise in order to achieve or continue to achieve fat loss or simply to maintain a healthy weight.

The City Caveman Plan is forging a 'new nutrition following', where real food becomes our first and only choice to positively affect our mental and physical wellbeing.

The City Caveman Plan, with its 10 grams of fat per meal, forced Mike to consume low saturated fat meals, and various studies have shown we can live better and longer by consuming a diet lower in such fats. To Mike's credit he has embraced this plan without a nutritional background and found that even in an urban environment, it is possible to source real food packed with antioxidants. These same antioxidants – found in carrots, broccoli, onions, garlic, beetroot, beans, cauliflower, figs, dates, apples, tomatoes, berries, grapes (the list is endless) and, of course, wine in moderation (after your forty days are over, of course) – help us not only to stay healthy, but they provide us with the best anti-ageing strategy available.

Lastly, enjoy your newfound energy and don't stress too much along the way. Every day is not going to be perfect, but that's okay because tomorrow brings new foods, new tastes, new intentions, improved nutrition and a better state of health!

I want you to be aware of what you're eating. It only takes a second to turn a can or a bottle around to read it's nutrition label. If you are reading it and thinking 'What the hell are those ingredients?', then take the hint: if too much of it is unknown, put it back! And if it reads like it's been cooked up in a chemist's lab, then it probably has! By learning a little about what's in your food, you will gain precious knowledge to help you accomplish your journey back to good health.

10

City Caveman Day Zero

I have learned from my travel adventures around the world that the journeys worth remembering are those that are fun, yet challenging. They have their ups and downs, but in the end they provide the best memories and build the most character. They're life changing, and you can never truly go back to your old self. I am hoping the City Caveman Plan will allow me to travel in a similar fashion. I am really looking forward to a fulfilling journey, to the learning process, to saying goodbye to my old, chubby self and to, hopefully, becoming a new person.

Back in 1998, I made my first trip out of the USA to live in London. While I thought I'd be mainly exploring Europe, I soon found myself meeting co-workers who were going to Russia, Australia, Tibet and all these places that I never thought I'd make it to in my life. It didn't take long before curiosity got the best of me, and I was flying solo for a hiking trip in Nepal.

It was undeniably the best adventure of my life. The culture, the people, the food, the hiking, the monkeys and the sight of Mount Everest; it was absolutely amazing. At one point during my trip I saw a group of men walking with their arms interlocked. It was no big deal, as I like to consider myself open-minded.

Days later, after hiking in The Himalayas (yes, there are 'easy' treks that even chubby chaps can go on), and having the most amazing group of Sherpas aide us with our gear, cooking and lodging, an Aussie traveller laughed at my recollection of the guys walking arm in arm in the city, and informed me that it was not a group of gay men in Kathmandu that I had seen, but rather, that was the way that they show friendship to each another; it was merely a cultural gesture to demonstrate mateship in Nepal.

During our hiking through the mountains, even though our Sherpas spoke zero-to-little English, I formed a friendly bond with one of the guys. Maybe it was because we had similar mannerisms, or maybe it was the way we laughed and smiled. I had my $200 hiking boots on and expensive gear to save me from the cold, while he was wearing thongs, jeans and carrying way more gear than should be allowed up and down those mountains! We were two chaps from very different cultures and backgrounds, but we still connected.

On our last day of hiking, I felt somebody come up from behind me, to interlock their arm around mine, just like I'd seen in Kathmandu. It was my Sherpa, and he was showing me that he thought of me as his friend, his mate. I was so touched. It's something I'll never forget.

But why this story?

Because I kind of hope that when someone reads about my City Caveman journey he or she will travel with me, the way I did in my experience in Nepal. Man or woman – I don't care – through the City Caveman Plan we will have a little connection, so you can think of me as interlocking your arm Nepalese-style, so we can become healthier together.

I know there are lots of people out there who are just like me; who need to make a change in order to save their life. And so, with all my heart and energy, I'm committing 100 per cent to the City Caveman Plan and hope that others can be inspired to make the same kind of change in themselves.

We have the entire travel map laid out, we have the Workout Plan, the Eating Plan and a goal to stay true to the Caveman Contract on the bathroom mirror. I promise to be honest about my journey and to never ever give up.

I hope my writing can make you laugh a bit, think a lot, and change your lifestyle with me…because I think by the end, it is going to be a whole lot better as we fully commit ourselves to our health and our (hopeful) new lives.

See you at the gym.

Mike the chubby Caveman.

11

City Caveman Days 1 to 10 – *Commitment*

Day 1. On Your Marks, Get Set...uh-oh!

It is hard to fail, but it is worse never to have tried to succeed.

– Theodore Roosevelt

I feel like I am 12 years old and about to board a roller-coaster. I'm excited yet very nervous.

And just as it is on a roller-coaster, I have the feeling of not truly knowing what lies ahead in my challenge, knowing there will be plenty of ups and downs, and just praying that things don't get too far off track.

A friend called this morning and asked 'What's new?' to which my response was 'Breakfast!' Yup...breakfast consumption was a new experience for me today, and I must say, it was damn good.

The City Caveman Plan is helping me understand that breakfast is the key to each day being a great one. It is the time of the day where I fill up my body with healthy food, so that it gives me back the energy I need to work out, feel good and get on with the physical demands of living.

Mentally, it felt great to start the day with a fresh, healthy fruit juice smoothie *and* it was damn tasty. Day 1 breakfast: successfully undertaken.

To the gym I went. Today was unlike the days of the past, because today I actually had a workout plan. It really is silly how many days I went to the gym with kind of a 'what should I do today?' attitude – no plan, no goal, no nothing. Today was definitely a new day.

I decided to assume an 'It's Game Day' approach to the workout, in a bid to motivate myself to focus on the actual exercise and really strive to achieve those results. I psyched myself up to just follow the plan and follow it hard. No perving, no time-wasting, just training. And guess what? It worked! I just hope my Game Day motivation doesn't wear off by Wednesday!

Surprisingly, my rope-jumping skills were pretty fresh from my high school basketball days, so I thought I was travelling pretty well through the workout. That was, until I caught a glimpse of myself in the mirror with my chub flying north and south in my too-tight t-shirt! My initial instinct was to curl up and die, but instead of crawling back into the darkness to hibernate, I decided to use that scary image to motivate me to skip even harder.

The 20 minutes of running was a challenge, but my Game Day mentality actually got me through it. Of course, then came the really hard part: weight training.

For me, opening the door to a doctor's office when a rectal exam is due is easier than entering a weight room. Weights and Mike just don't naturally mix because, traditionally, my insecurities are rife when I am surrounded by fit folks doing what they do best. But, Game Day had to prevail, so as badly as I wanted to race out of there, I summoned my courage, sucked in my gut, pumped out my man boobs and stuck to the Plan.

I always feel like people are staring and judging me while in the weight room, but you know what I realise? My time in the gym has nothing to do with anyone other than me, and I need to really understand that my mission is unique to me.

Caveman Tip:

Your journey to better health is unique to you.

I wish that I could magically wake up tomorrow to find my body is in the shape I want it to be; but, since that's not going to happen, today I will be happy with my single, baby step towards improving my health and life.

Day 1. Done and dusted.

Annie says: *It's the start of the City Caveman Plan! How exciting. I love the starts of things: relationships, journeys, workout schedules. It's a time when you are most in touch with the realm of possibilities that could come from your efforts. Your energy is at its highest and you are motivated by the thought of achieving your goal. As Mike describes, it feels like getting on a roller-coaster: scary but thrilling at the same time. Every journey starts with the first step and, today, Mike took his first step.*

Mike is enjoying the natural high that comes with starting a new journey. As a fitness professional, I know that there will be many uphill battles to face along the way, including both psychological and physical challenges. Despite the marketing jargon, there are no magic pills or easy-fix remedies, except to keep focused on the end goal and to commit to following your plan. I am happy that Mike had a mental high today, and I hope it continues, because undoubtedly, along the way he will fall prone to a few mental lows, which is natural when we are in the process of fighting unhealthy habits. Mike's challenge is similar to a marathon run; you start strong, have highs and lows throughout the journey, yet at the end you can laugh, cry and throw your arms up into the air in victory because you reached your goal!

Mind and body change will not happen overnight, and I have informed Mike of this. Yes, I know he was being cheeky when he wished Mother Nature could give him a new body overnight, but it is important to remember that any short-term results are likely to stay short-term results. I urge you to simply follow the Plan day by day, and you can look at what's evolved when you reach Day 41.

As Mike described, feeling scared or intimidated to walk into a gym is very common for new exercisers. Being surrounded by fit people can be scary, but remember that they were once new to the gym too! So, instead of letting this fear stop you from working out, try and be inspired by these fit people. They weren't always fit, and they still have insecurities like you do, albeit in a different context. The mind is a very powerful tool, so spend some time visualising where you want your mind and body to be at the end of forty days. A golfer, for example, visualises his shot from the fairway landing two metres from the pin; a pole vaulter visualises herself clearing the bar, while an AFL player sees himself putting the 40-metre kick through the 6-point goal. If you set your mind to it, you can do it; visualise your new healthy life and new fit body, and it can be yours.

Day 2. Food Frustration

> *Laughter and tears are both responses to frustration and exhaustion . . . I myself prefer to laugh, since there is less cleaning up to do afterward.*
>
> – Kurt Vonnegut

Day 2 started with an early 40-minute run on the treadmill, which I initially didn't really know how I would manage. But I understood that having a workout plan meant a 40-minute run should see me running for 40 minutes! I had to hold myself accountable and, while it was not easy, and I did take quite a few water breaks, eventually I made it through. When I think about going to the gym *without* a set goal or workout plan, well, I don't even know why I bothered! I can see now how creating a plan and following it through really works.

After the workout was breakfast. Now nothing shits a chubby chap more than having a bad food day, and today was one of those days. According to my Caveman breakfast menu, it was *egg-white omelette day*, which made it the first day in my entire life that I would eat a healthy omelette. Historically, my choice of omelette was laden with cheese, ham, bacon, salt and an abundance of tomato sauce. So, for me to go from 'hangover omelette' to 'energy omelette' was definitely a change.

I had planned to have an egg-white omelette with mushrooms, red pepper, a little spice and tomato accompanied by a big fresh squeezed orange juice, however, the 40-minute cardio workout, along with the soreness from yesterday's weight session left me feeling so spent that cooking was out of the question. I decided dining out would be my best bet, so I legged it over to a nearby Austrian restaurant. Austria was the choice of the day, given that my girlfriend is Austrian, but trying to enquire about a special order using only 'white eggs' proved to be too difficult for the cooks to comprehend. So home I went, officially turning *egg-white omelette* day into *fruit smoothie day*.

Unfortunately, my food frustration continued through the day when, on my way home, I passed a kebab shop. Now, I LOVE the smell of kebab shops. The meat, the chips – the smell is like a magnet to me. However, reminding myself that Cavemen never saw cone-shaped, processed meat like the kebab shops create, I knew that my only option was to walk on by in the hopes of finding some fresh, lean chicken like the Cavemen would have done. And so I bid farewell to my favourite little shop of horror.

Changing patterns is very difficult. From the way we get to work, to our daily TV viewing, to our eating habits – we are creatures of habit. My pre-Caveman eating pattern was to consume the most convenient, tastiest meal or snack that I could find, regardless of its nutritional content. I do think that one of my greatest challenges in the coming thirty-eight days will be to overturn my existing eating habits and instincts.

Snack time is such a ritual…a habit…a must. I am so conditioned to opening my cupboards and refrigerator to grab a cheeky bag of crisps or a sugary treat. It's so hard to stop snooping and sniffing around the kitchen cabinets looking for something to eat. This caveman is battling – battling hard.

Caveman Tip:

Don't stock the naughty stuff at home, and then you can't be tempted to eat it!

My run was damn good today, but changing my diet and avoiding the naughty stuff is going to be a LOT more difficult than I initially envisioned.

Day 2 is done. And so three more Caveman boxes are ticked off my list on my mirror. I am 5 per cent of the way there.

Annie says: *The food issue is the thing that most people find hardest to change in their lifestyles. If you are struggling with your weight and health as Mike is, you are probably accustomed to using food for pleasure. Unfortunately, that usually equates to eating too many fatty, sugar-dense foods. On a global scale, we have evolved to eating junky, fatty food because it is so cheap to purchase, profitable to produce and convenient to obtain. Also, it is challenging to eat healthy when you are eating out; workdays are getting longer and more stressful, so a naughty meal with dessert can be an easy way to stimulate one's senses to provide pleasure during the day.*

As Mike found, there can be a healthy eating barrier. For example, a lot of restaurants wouldn't know what an egg-white omelette is, let alone how to make it. Although many healthy salad options are popping up around Australia, we still have a way to go regarding fresh, fast foods.

So to Mike, on Day 2, I am recommending he avoids the restaurant industry for forty days as best as he can, remembering that unless he cooks it, he can't be certain of its contents. After all, the crux of the City Caveman Plan is to return to the Caveman days, where food was fresh, simple and tasty without preservatives, additives or flavouring. And in order to accurately watch your fat, sodium and sugar intake, you really do need to prepare it in your kitchen.

So Mike, you successfully completed two out of forty days. Please do not look at this as a prison sentence, just keep ticking off those boxes on your Caveman Contract and enjoy the satisfaction of knowing that you battled and won on that particular day. We all need that daily satisfaction because it will serve to propel and motivate you into the next day, as well as holding you accountable for the days to come. That said however, DO NOT become a day-counter. In fact, please do your best to NOT count the days at all. We have committed to a 40-day plan, so try to keep your focus on the end of the forty days, rather than clock-watch every day. To help with this, try seeking out new mental and physical challenges, because this will help you vary your routine and contribute to helping you adjust to change. And rather than thinking you've done two out of forty days, look at it as having just thirty-eight days left of fun, healthy challenges!

It is only natural that the body and taste buds will have a tantrum as you introduce new things to them. But, eventually, your taste buds will adjust and, before you know it, you will actually be looking forward to those healthy, tasty meals! Of course, temptation will always be in your face, and if you need to substitute an egg-white omelette with a healthy smoothie, so be it; just don't substitute it with an egg and bacon croissant that has 40 grams of fat! In the past, Mike would have made an unconscious decision to indulge in whatever he wanted, but with the City Caveman Plan, he now makes conscious decisions NOT to indulge. Such a shift in behaviour is a difficult task, but one that needs to be made in order to create a healthy lifestyle forever.

Day 3. A Workout Date with The Boss

> *I've always found that the speed of the boss is the speed of the team.*
>
> – Lee Iacocca

Today was a big day: my first workout with Annie. A little nervous, a little excited. A leg workout was on the menu. At this point in time I'd hoped that menu would contain a roast beef sandwich with caramelised onions and mozzarella cheese, but, sadly…legs. D'oh.

My first lesson of the day was that I discovered how anger can enhance a workout. If you're angry at the boss, take it out at the gym. If you've got spousal issues, hit the weights, hard! If the traffic report says your commute home will be one-and-a-half hours longer, run harder on the treadmill to work away that angst. For me, I was furious with the gym because on Day 1 of the Caveman Plan, I actually lost my pass to the gym.

I'm an idiot. I'll wear that. Having no pockets in my shorts, I was bound to leave my pass on a machine or on the ground somewhere during my workout, but what really pissed me off was the fact that to be issued with a new pass (a new piece of plastic) was going to cost me $20.

Being able to exorcise my frustrations and anger via my workout was very timely. I really like Annie's no bullshit style; she knows I'm chubby, and she knows *I know* I'm chubby, so we can just get down to the business of improving the situation. All in all, the leg workout sucked, which means the chubby chap hated it, and the personal trainer loved it.

As I left the gym, walking down the stairs made my legs shake. They were so worn out that I still feel the soreness some eight hours later. Thank you Annie… I think.

Tonight I had two food epiphanies. The first had to do with pasta. Prior to my Caveman challenge, pasta night was usually a small pyramid of garlic toast, egg fettuccine noodles drowned in creamy pasta sauce with bacon bits and a stack of parmesan cheese piled over the top. Total fat grams? Infinity. Seriously, who knows? I once heard that the two unhealthiest servings on any menu are pasta with fettuccine Alfredo sauce (exactly what I just described), and eggs with hollandaise sauce (another favourite hangover cure of mine).

Given that Cavemen did not know about Alfredo sauce back in their time, I was forced to try an alternative pasta dish. In one pan I cooked fresh mushrooms, pepper, onion and a full tomato. I topped it with one cup full of organic pasta sauce, then dropped in a few prawns and scallops. Then, rather than my usual huge helping of egg fettuccine noodles, I grabbed just one handful of wholemeal penne pasta. Of course, my initial thought was 'There's no way this will be enough pasta,' yet after adding fresh, healthy tomato sauce, tonnes of great veggies, prawns and scallops, I had an enormous bowl of healthy, tasty pasta which, if I do say so myself, was quite delicious! My discovery of the day was that fresh and healthy pasta *can* be made with very few fat grams, and if *I* could pull it off, then anyone can!

My second epiphany occurred as I was pulling the veggies out of the fridge. For the first time in a very long time, I actually felt good about what was in my refrigerator. Traditionally stocked with beer, fizzy drinks, wine, chocolate, cheeses, vodka and other assorted bad-for-you goodies, my Caveman change now saw my fridge bursting at the seams with freshly squeezed juices, fish, salads, skim milk, berries, apples, tomatoes, onions and lots more healthy fare. I realised that it actually feels fantastic to open it up and see fresh, instead of processed foods.

Caveman Tip:

Caveman creativity in the kitchen is great for the mind, tastebuds and waistline.

Day 3: So far so good? Actually, so far so great!

***Annie says**: Ah, legs day. I love training legs; it's challenging and sometimes painful but the rewards include having sexy legs and a toned butt, and who wouldn't want that? Funnily enough, however, there seems to be a universal neglect of leg workouts by so many people in the gyms. As a fitness professional, I can only plead that everyone performs a well-balanced workout from head to toe. That includes keeping a healthy mind, working on your chest, arms, back, shoulders AND legs! I equate working out legs to baking a loaf of Grandma's Christmas Banana Bread. She did not just bake half of the loaf and leave the other half out of the oven to go uncooked, did she? Don't let your legs be the uncooked, under-worked part of your body. Your workouts, like life, are all about balance.*

Mike continues to call himself names and indulge in negative self-talk. However, like many of us, Mike is too tough on himself. It's really important in this process to encourage ourselves to achieve the end goal, rather than keep feeding ourselves with negative comments. Also, by focusing on the negative, we take away energy we could be using to make the positive changes we desire. Our energy is best invested in what we want to become in the future.

Yes, we did use Mike's anger today to help him have an awesome workout. We both walked out of there on shaky, wobbly legs, actually; it really is rewarding to experience that endorphin rush after a legs workout. You go into it all hyped up and, for the rest of the day, you feel relaxed and hungry.

Now, I should have made this point on Day 1 when Mike began weight training, but I will make it now:

WEIGHT TRAINING IS ESSENTIAL FOR MEN AND WOMEN.

I think the biggest misconception of working out comes from women thinking that they will get big and bulky if they start using weights. But this is a fallacy. In order to lose fat and/or firm up, weights are an absolute necessity as they increase metabolism, which means you will actually continue to burn fat long after your workout has ended and your legs have stopped shaking! The Caveman Workout Plan is designed for both men and women. Cardio may keep one slim, but it's the weights that add the tone and shape that truly define one's figure.

Day 4. Holy Shhhhh...Soreness Prevails!

> *No pain? No gain.*
>
> – Author unknown

Ouch. I am sore, and I realised it before I was even fully awake this morning.

Today, when my alarm clock went off, the first thing I knew was that I was unbelievably, amazingly sore from my leg workout with Annie; so much so that I actually had trouble getting out of bed, sitting on the toilet and walking down stairs. Everything I did that involved movement below the waist was a chore because of the tenderness.

And to make matters worse, on a full morning train, I had to sit on what we Americans call the 'half-assed seat' of the train. It's that seat where one butt cheek is right on the seam of where the seat starts. Anyway, that seam hit my right butt cheek, which forced me to let out an attention-pulling 'ohhhhhhhhhh' noise in front of all those people. You know you have sore muscles when the seam of a bloody seat cushion causes you pain equal to that of a stab wound. This was not going to be my best-ever Thursday.

Of course, on the positive side, soreness means my muscles had a good workout, which is a good thing. And given that the soreness from Monday's workout has now disappeared, I can assume this pain will also disappear before too long. I also gained some perspective when I watched a documentary where a double amputee man (with a bad case of high-altitude laryngitis) successfully climbed Mount Everest with his two prosthetic limbs. It's amazing how a man missing the bottom half of both parts of his legs has the mental capacity and physical energy to climb one of the world's most treacherous mountains! I figured that if he could climb the highest peak in the world with two non-working legs, I could somehow cope with a case of sore legs!

Caveman Tip:

Inspiration is everywhere – find yours, and turn it into energy.

Unfortunately, despite my sore legs, it was cardio day with some additional abdominal work. Of course, I whined like a goof about it to Annie on the phone, begging her to explain how in the world, if I could hardly sit on the toilet, I could run for 40 minutes at the gym? I really didn't know how I could complete a full workout when I was feeling so sore. Even the warm-up stretch felt nearly impossible. Annie was slightly sympathetic and told me to do my best, saying that even 60 per cent of normal running would be a good effort for the day. I liked this logic.

After limping to the gym, I proceeded to the workout room for my stretch. The tightness of my leg muscles felt as tight as a fully extended bungy cord with Rosie O'Donnell dangling off the end! My warm-up stretching was a painful, no-fun task today. Each stretch was this slow pull-pull-pull on my muscle, although, interestingly, I couldn't decide if it was painful or pleasurable – regardless, it was necessary for my run.

The 40-minute schedule had been reduced to 24 minutes, thanks to Annie's leniency. I expected the treadmill to feel like one of those leg-torture machines, but I was sort of wrong; sort of. The soreness was definitely present, but once I got started, once I got my body moving, things started to feel surprisingly… normal. Mentally, I managed to push through the diminishing ache, all the while telling myself to 'just get it done'. And so that's what I did. For the full 40 minutes.

Now, before you stand up for the ovation, I need to tell you, I did skip the abdominal workout! There was just NO chance I was sitting on two sore butt cheeks to do some abdominal work, so I decided that I'd make it up on Friday. Sure, my 40-minute run was slow, but powering through the pain certainly gave this Caveman a victory over the day's battle.

Annie says: *I've been waiting for the soreness to overwhelm Mike. I'd been hesitant to warn him about what was headed his way, because I did not want him backing off the intensity of his training in these first few days. Delayed onset of muscle soreness (also called DOMS) is not like a few hairs out of place that can be fixed with some hair gel; there is no quick fix, no easy cure. When muscle soreness is present, you just have to work through it.*

I view soreness as a good sign because if you have pushed your muscles hard enough, they will be sore the next day, and this means you have improved your strength and muscle tone. The only real cure to combat this soreness is to make sure you eat plenty of protein and drink lots of water to compensate for the muscle breakdown.

I am really pleased that Mike didn't give up entirely after his first hit of post-workout pain. I was very proud that he went for his run even though he felt like having a couch day!

Now, let me share a little secret with you: The trick to beating soreness is getting to the gym and starting your workout.

Once you start, you'll usually keep going, especially if you have a goal in mind. I think Mike knew he had Caveman boxes to check off at night, and he did not want to put 60 per cent of a tick next to the 40-minute run box. I knew that if I could just get Mike to the gym and running (by telling him he could do 60 per cent) that he would end up completing 100 per cent once he started. It is difficult, but if you are not in the mood to workout (and let's face it, that might be a common state to be in for many of you), then commit to going and working out for just 10 minutes. Then, if you still feel like you can't do it, go ahead and go home early. Nine times out of ten though, once you get started, you will complete the task at hand in its entirety.

Day 5. Healthy Battles

> *You cannot dream yourself into a character; you must hammer and forge yourself into one.*
>
> – James A. Froude

I developed a very important mindset today. On my way to the gym this morning (hell, on my way to anywhere), I came across a doughnut shop. Now, of course, doughnuts are not part of the City Caveman food plan, so *I forced myself to hurry on by.* This might not sound like a really big deal, but I disagree. I think it is a big deal, because it made me realise something that I think could carry me through my 35 remaining days. It made me realise that:

Every day is filled with little battles. Whether it is battling against drinking that beer, staying away from the fish and chip shop, or finishing the final minute of that cardio workout, every day will present me with new and repeated small battles that I can choose to win or to lose. I am determined to win.

I know that if I can win each of those smaller battles during my forty days, then I can win the war! Forty days can seem like a large, intimidating chunk of time, but if I break it down battle-by-battle and victory-by-victory, then my motivation to keep winning can only keep getting bigger.

Each day, I probably walk past fifty fast food outlets, bars, ice cream shops and so on. By looking at my old eating habits, I probably gave in and indulged in thirty to forty of those unhealthy options every week. From buying a fast food meal to a late night chocolate bar to an unnecessary soft drink, I gave in way too much. Yet, the City Caveman Plan has zero room for such selections, so to win this war, I need to go from thirty to forty deviant choices to ZERO. I will battle, and it will be difficult – but I know I can do it.

Of course my battles are not limited to just food or alcohol offerings; they also encompass the physical battles, especially since those workouts do leave my body quite sore. Physically, I was still feeling quite rough today, so I was faced with two options: skip the workout and couch it, or battle through the pain and complete my run and weights day as the Plan dictates. I chose the latter. Again, it was a slow but steady run to start, and I just kept telling myself: If I win the battles, both mentally and physically, then I will create change.

It sounds great in theory, but to be honest, part of me expects that I will hit the wall sooner or later. At some point I think I will falter with a night out on the drink or a pizza indulgence. This negative thought makes me feel quite disappointed with myself. Here I am taking on the City Caveman Plan and feeling good about my step-by-step progress, yet part of me also still expects to fail on some level. What's that about? It's crap to feel like that. I guess perhaps this self-doubt arises from all the old patterns of excuses that I used to make before I was a Caveman. Perhaps what used to be 'delay' of making change has now been replaced with 'doubt' that I can actually succeed.

Today was full of doubt and battles; not only with cheeky food offerings and painful workouts, but today I battled my first Friday night as a City Caveman.

Friday nights are traditionally spent in a bar after work. I happen to live in an inner-city suburb, which is rife with beautiful waterside bars that are filled with temptation and that are open to all hours of the night. However, as a City Caveman, Friday nights are now no longer for drinking.

Even so, after my first week of Caveman living, a slightly sympathetic side within figured that perhaps I deserve a few congratulatory drinks, for having done so well so far, and so I caught up with my mate, Marty. He is recently single, so we headed to a popular bar that had lots of beautiful 'scenery' (i.e. women!).

Marty shouted my first *drink*: a mineral water with fresh lime. No doubt, this was a first in my lifetime; ordering a water at 7pm on a Friday, in a pumping bar. I started to think I might well be a certifiably insane City Caveman.

I felt like a square peg trying to fit into a round hole, sitting there in the middle of Sydney's busiest social venue on a Friday night, sipping water. And so, after two waters and a quick chat with Marty, my Friday evening was over.

I knew the time would come where I'd have to socialise without drinking alcohol, but to be honest, I wasn't mentally prepared for it. If the truth be known, I can't actually recall the last time I went for more than two days without an alcoholic drink.

Food. Alcohol. Soreness. Facing the weights. This week it has been all about saying 'yes' to the good and 'no' to the bad. It is harder than I thought, but I am battling. And so far I am winning.

Caveman Tip:

Be conscious of your battles. Face them head on. Win. And you will create change.

Annie says: *Mike mentioned the self-doubt he has regarding his successful completion of the Caveman Plan. This uncertainty is extremely normal behaviour because he has spent so many years, until now, conditioning his mind, his taste buds and his body to act and react certain ways in response to those cheeky foods and alcohol nights. The only way to combat those thoughts and minimise the frequency at which they occur, is to stick with the Plan. We are on Day 5, and I think Mike has a pretty good support network in the daily Workout and Eating Plans, my encouragement, and his Caveman checklist, which acts like a third person to keep him on track, motivated and accountable for his daily actions.*

Even while he is successfully changing his behavioural patterns, self-doubt will linger because, mentally, he has not yet fully changed. All I can do to support him during these moments of weakness is encourage him to battle, to win and to stay positive. Very soon, that self-doubt will be gone and replaced with a healthy confidence that will make the remaining City Caveman Plan days go by very, very smoothly.

I like Mike's line of thinking in terms of his battles. I like that he can objectively see that there are battles that must be won. Recognising that 'Yes, this is a battle, and this is a time where I must say no so I can win it' is a great thought process to have. The battles will continue, but by consciously knowing that it is 'battle time', there is a much, much higher likelihood of saying 'no' to that doughnut or bottle of beer.

The thing is, everybody who is overweight and starting out on a fat-loss plan will have to fight that little voice in their head that says 'stay in bed instead of exercising', or 'eat that doughnut instead of a piece of fruit', and 'junk food tastes great'. With persistence and time, Mike will soon hear himself saying, 'I love feeling fit and healthy', 'I love having more energy', and 'I love the way I look in my jeans'. And one day, he will actually enjoy his workouts so much that he will genuinely want to go for a run or do a weight training session. Similarly, he will prefer to eat a healthy salad and grilled fish over a hot dog, because he'll prefer the taste and he'll love how good he feels after eating it. Once that change takes effect in his psyche, there is no stopping how fit and healthy he can become.

So Mike, well done on winning a week full of battles! I am confident you will be just as good a soldier in Week 2.

Day 6. The Good, the Bad and the Ugly

> *What if this is as good as it gets?*
>
> – Melvin Udall (Jack Nicholson) in *As Good as It Gets*

The process of motivating myself, having good workouts and noticing a few good changes was a nice wave that I enjoyed riding for the first five days. But that wave ended today. Today was a true mix of the good, the bad and the ugly.

The Good

Saturday morning arrived, and I was off to a great start, largely due to the fact I actually got a good night's sleep. The lack of Friday night drinks may have been tough on me psychologically, but physically, my body thanked me many times over! I slept soundly all night, and I woke up feeling fresh and healthy, with clear eyes and a very clear head. It's quite a change from the norm over the past few years. I could not have felt better.

So, I headed straight to the gym for my Saturday morning run. Afterwards, I felt absolutely golden. I know I am only six days into my City Caveman Plan, but I can only describe my clear head as ecstasy. It feels as though someone turned the lights on inside me. It felt great.

Still feeling thirsty, on my way home I stopped by the local fruit and veggie shop for a bottle of water. I entered the shop, and my conversation went just like this:

'Hi there. Can I please have a water?'

'Yes, sure. $2 please.'

'Thanks. Oh wait (spotting wheatgrass in the background)... ummm, what's that wheatgrass stuff like?'

'Well, it is very healthy.'

'Ha ha. That must mean it tastes like crap!'

'Most think so, yes.'

'Why do people drink it then?'

'One shot has the nutrient value of 2 kilograms of veggies.'

'Wow, potent. Did you know Homer Simpson made a wheatgrass mixed with vodka cocktail called 'The Lawnmower'? Did you see that episode?'

(*Looks puzzled*) 'No.'
'Ummm, what if I put it in a smoothie. Would it taste better?'
'It would ruin the taste of the smoothie.'
'Strong stuff then. Okay, I will just do the shot then, and chase it with the water.'
'The water won't help you. You will definitely need a juice chaser.'
'Yikes. I'm still game. I will have a fresh orange juice as well, please.'

I was about to consume grass. And let it be known that I have a bad history with this stuff. No, not *smoking* grass, but *mowing* grass. When I was in my early teens, the horrid chore of mowing the lawn was left up to me. I disliked it so much that I left it undone week after week, until Mum eventually gave up asking me. So we stopped watering the lawn altogether and, as a result, we were the only family on the street whose yard was covered with a dead, yellow-coloured hay.

Holding my green gunk and orange juice chaser, I finally took a whiff of my wheatgrass shot. And guess what? It smelled exactly like the grass that I never mowed!

Amazingly, I *enjoyed* my first wheatgrass shot. The taste is hard to describe because, wheatgrass does not taste like anything else; it tastes exactly as it smells – like grass. Sure, I wouldn't mix it with vodka during social events but, if such a grassy, magic potion packs a punch with so many nutrients, I could certainly stomach it a couple of times a week for health's sake. I shall mark down another healthy change for Caveman Mike.

Funny how I refused to mow grass, and now 20 years later I'm drinking it! Strange, but good times.

Coming home I was in bright spirits. I had a great workout and, according to the fruity dreadlock chap, I had also consumed the equivalent of two kilograms of healthy veggies in one little plastic shot glass. Just a week ago I was accustomed to alcohol-fuelled sleep, shocking hangovers, greasy food, ineffective workouts and overall laziness. But today, I have great sleep, healthy food, fabulous exercise and energy that lasts all day.

The Bad

Prior to pressing PLAY on the *As Good as It Gets* DVD that I hired for my night in, I thought I would do a little Caveman monitoring. All week I had avoided jumping on the scales to see if I'd made progress; but tonight, I was feeling good, so I thought: what better way to check my progress, than to don those same jeans that I wore in my original photo? Let the good times roll!

What a bad, bad idea that turned out to be!

As high as my spirits were all day Saturday, they dropped just as low at the first sight of my 'new' photos. And shame on me for even taking them and thinking that I had undergone some miraculous physical transformation in only six days! The damn jeans were just as impossible to button, and I looked just as fat and chubby as I did in them six days ago.

Compounding what was now a crap mood was the fact that I had no idea how to set the camera timer, so I actually had to set up a mirror for me to be able to take the stupid photos. How embarrassing! There I was, holding the camera toward a mirror, all the while posing, being chubby and taking self-portraits – how sad! I threw the jeans straight into the bin. They're gone, and with them went my newfound confidence and all my aspirations of a nice body.

> *The good workout, the bad idea to think I had transformed over night, and the ugly photos – what a day it was.*

So, it was a hard lesson to learn but I realised there are definitely no one-week shortcuts, and I should definitely expect that not every Caveman day will be a good one.

Caveman Tip:

Change takes time. Stay committed, and be patient.

The Ugly

Let's hope these photos are not as good as it gets!

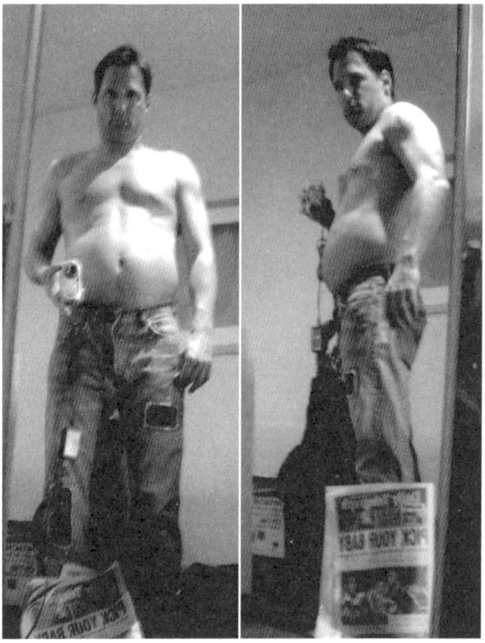

Annie says: *Poor Mike. At the risk of sounding clichéd, these things do happen. We knew these forty days would be a roller-coaster and, unfortunately, it happened to him on this particular Saturday.*

As for trying on his jeans after only six days: BAD MOVE! It's as bad as jumping on the scales and weighing yourself. Don't ever do it again! In fact, until Day 40 arrives, if you can help it, don't weigh, monitor, measure or judge yourself. Yes, it is difficult, because we all want confirmation that we are making progress, but this is a huge mistake that many people who are trying to lose weight make. They expect instant results and, when the scale is still the same or they look the same in the mirror, they get discouraged and give up. Real, sustainable fat loss is gradual, and while it's fantastic that you are feeling like significant changes have taken place mentally, it may take longer to reflect the same level of achievement physically. I am happy with the emotional changes Mike has achieved after his first week. The physical transformation will also arrive with time.

Another reason to stay off the scales is because if you weigh yourself in the early days, you may actually weigh more than you used to. This can lead to depression or feelings of failure, which can then lead you to give up the Plan. But, what you need to understand is that muscle weighs more than fat so you can actually weigh more on the scales, even though you're actually becoming healthier. Remember, your quest for good health has you on a mission to achieve FAT loss, not WEIGHT loss.

The other mistake people make is to go on starvation diets and, unfortunately, bookstores and the internet are loaded with these 'lose weight quickly' fads. Starvation diets break down muscles and slow your metabolism. And this is why the dieter will put all the weight (and usually more!) right back on, once they start eating normally again. When it's starved, and the muscles start to break down, the body has so little muscle to burn fat that when food is eaten again, it stores it as fat, in anticipation of being starved again.

So, if you remember anything from this book, remember this: the best way to lose body fat is to regularly exercise and eat healthy food. I do not like the term 'weight loss' because you need to be careful what type of weight you are losing. For if it is muscle loss, then in the long term, you are actually taking two steps backwards in terms of overall health. What we need to aim for is FAT loss and lean muscle gain, not WEIGHT loss.

Day 7. Mother's Day…Off

No rest is worth anything except the rest that is earned.

– Jean Paul

Sunday, Sunday – City Caveman day off! Well, not fully a day off, as I still have to adhere to the eating plan, but I am giving my statuesque body a day off from training. After another grand night of sleep, I have semi-forgotten about last night's fatty-photo blunder. Well, not fully, since I just mentioned it, but I'm not going to give up and get drunk over it; I will just continue on.

Today is Mother's Day, so I spoke with Mum this morning, who is back in Arizona. I miss her. She was here just two weeks ago, and we had a great time together.

With no workout planned for today, and with Mom living too far away to visit, it really was a day off for me. So, I invited Annie out for a friendly Mother's Day brunch by the beach. We met down at Coogee Beach, and Annie was running late (ahhhhem – if I was late, I would have to run extra sprints as a punishment. Annie being late? I have to wait. I guess being the chubby student has made me the powerless one in this arrangement!).

To kill some time, I did a light beachside run and then took a people-watching walk up and down Coogee Beach. I popped my head into the local pub. It was 11am, and twenty people were inside smoking and drinking away. 11am – apparently it's never too early to breathe in some cigarette smoke and have a few drinks! I felt good about my Caveman aspirations. I'd originally moved to Sydney to enjoy the outdoors, lead a clean life and improve my lifestyle, but in reality I was living a life that would more likely find me in that pub with those other people. I decided right there and then that I would never be *that* guy in that bar ever again.

Annie and I went on a lazy walk with Annie's son, Hunter, from Coogee Beach to Bronte Beach and back. This beachfront walk is one of the geographical highlights of Sydney, winding up stairs, around cliff faces, and leading to numerous beaches and cafes.

During the walk, I made a promise to never let myself get to the point where I could not do this walk. This walk really symbolises the reason why I moved to Australia – to be around the sun and the outdoors – yet I see so many people missing out on the chance to experience Australia in all its glory because of their health (or lack thereof!).

Just last month I spoke with a tourist visiting from my home city of Chicago. He and his wife were around 38 years old and both a bit on the hefty side (that is being polite). When they asked what they should do while in the Bondi area, I told them about the 40-minute walk. He and his wife exchanged that 'I know what you are thinking and you know what I am thinking' look that couples have, after which he said, 'Ah, my wife isn't a good walker, so we'll probably have to give it a miss.'

Not a good walker? NOT A GOOD WALKER? I can understand she may not be a good footballer, or a good basketball player, or a good javelin thrower, but not a good walker?

It's these sorts of incidents that keep me inspired to continue on the City Caveman journey.

Caveman Tip:

Stay focused on changing bad health into good. There's too much to see and experience in life to let poor health dictate what you can and can't experience.

I am only one week into the Plan, but for now I am starting to feel less like that guy at the bar and a bit more like a healthy person. And while I accept that my photos don't yet portray how I am feeling, I will continue. I am proud to admit that for week one, this City Caveman has fared pretty damn well.

Annie says*: Mike went for a run on his day off! I am so impressed, even if it was just a light jog. Add to that our beach walk, and he earned gold stars today! Not only does he get stars for the extra effort, but also for spending it with me on Mother's Day! As a single mother, the day was looking like a 'stay at home and feel sorry for myself' one, because I don't have a partner to spoil me, but Mike saved me from attending a self-pity party and, instead, we had a great time filled with yummy, healthy food, great company and a very pleasant beachside walk in the sun.*

Regarding my tardiness, I have to apologise, but infants are very hard to predict and organise according to a clock. They are awake when you want them to sleep, asleep when you need them to be awake and when they do fall asleep, you never know how long they will stay asleep for. They're as puzzling as a Rubik's Cube, although 1,000 times more fun!

Mike thinks the City Caveman lifestyle is hard with the ups and downs (wait till he has his first child; it will seem like a walk in the park). And if my lateness allowed Mike to have a peek in the pub and learn another Caveman lesson about how he does NOT want his life to be, then I'm not actually too sorry at all!

I am excited about Mike's upcoming second Caveman week. I think he is in the right mindset to keep pushing it this week. He has followed the food plan, worked out quite hard, and he has battled the battles and won. Psychologically, he is on a winning streak and, as we all now know, if you can win the mental battle, the physical change will soon follow. He is still not quite there, but I sense he is starting to say 'goodbye' to much of his old lifestyle and 'hello' to a new, healthier life. It just takes time, but after a full week, I can see very clearly that Mike has the motivation and willpower to keep progressing well.

Cheers to us mothers on Mother's Day, and cheers to you Mike. Well done on your successful first week as a City Caveman.

Day 8. The Answer is Staring Right Back at Me

> *There are no shortcuts to any place worth going.*
>
> – Beverly Sills

The dreaded Monday weights day. I don't know if this part will ever get easier. I still feel a bit intimidated walking into that weight room, and the gym today was full of extra fit folks strutting their stuff. But, screw it. Who cares, right? It's not about them, it's about me. And that mentality is just another battle that I will win, eventually.

I battled through my bicep, tricep and shoulder workout pretty well, fighting off the weights room insecurities. Is it easier than it was in week one? Apart from knowing where the weights are located in the room, not really. The exercises are still new, and my muscles have not grown overnight, so my workout has certainly *not* become significantly easier…yet.

I did have one extra victory today though: I think I felt that 'gym buzz' that people talk about. Some runners speak of having 'runner's high', and today my training session really got my blood pumping, causing me to have a little skip in my step on the way home. And you know what? My workout buzz actually stayed with me throughout the entire day.

Tonight I hit a Caveman cooking milestone: I used a wok! And I loved it so much that I adopted it as my new favourite kitchen accessory; my own, personal City Caveman cooking pot.

I also did a bit of housekeeping, which led me to discover some sort of vitamin/diet pill/fat metaboliser that I had purchased a few months back thinking it was going to be the magical cure to my chubbiness. What a waste of money. Hundreds of millions of dollars are spent every year on diet pills and other associated shit. Even though I *know* there is no 'quick fix,' I still went out and bought into a gimmick, just because I wanted the end goal without having to actually contribute to the process, and the proof is right there in my own medicine cabinet!

Isn't it amazing how we look for the easy way out and the shortcuts? And, of course, the diet pills are just the beginning. From wacky diets to easy ab workout apparatuses to the ultimate – plastic surgery to remove fat, lift some part of the body, or smooth out some sort of wrinkle. And then there's the risk of taking these unknown diet pills or undergoing crazy surgeries, and the outrageous expense!

Caveman Tip:

The answer to a healthier life is the cheapest option of all: healthy eating, lower alcohol intake and good workouts.

The answer to good health is not found with a scalpel and it is definitely not found in the bathroom medicine cabinet! The only person who can make the change is staring right back at me in that mirror!

We live in a 'now' culture. Are you sick? Got a cold? No worries at all, take this pill. Are you hungry? Want a pizza? Make a call and it's at your doorstep in 30 minutes. Big body? Call the doctor for a super-duper weight loss pill! So many things are promoted as being obtainable *right now*, and health and fitness are no different. But, with the obesity rate in Australia climbing to 60 per cent, I think it's pretty obvious that if there is an easy fix, it's not working in the long term.

So, as I take these pills located behind the medicine cabinet and flush them down the toilet, I will discard my dreams and thoughts that there is an easy fix to fat loss and fitness. And I'll soldier on with the remaining thirty-two days of the City Caveman Plan to make it work for me and hopefully change my life forever.

Annie says: *Mike's workouts are not getting any easier, but this is good news! Think about it – workouts are never meant to be easy! And if they are, then you should actually be forcing yourself to put in more effort by increasing the weight or furthering your distance. By upping the intensity of your workouts you will push yourself to the next level of fitness.*

With Mike being in Week 2, I'd still expect the weights workouts to feel just as hard as they were last week, with the only key difference being that soreness levels have lessened. Then, once that soreness cycle disappears, your body is free to really push hard to give 100 per cent on every exercise. It takes a lot of concentration to give 100 per cent, but I implore you to do so because it will turn you into a fat-burning machine!

As Mike says, taking the easy way toward improved health is exactly the kind of thinking that makes someone overweight. Taking the 'easy path' in life is the path that leads you to buy fast food because you don't have time to prepare a meal.

It also leads you to lie on the couch or sit in front of a computer to 'veg out' rather than going for a walk, a bike ride or a swim.

There is no easy fix to becoming healthy, yet there is a very easy solution – healthy eating, moderate drinking and effective workouts.

See? It really is simple.

So, instead of taking the so-called easy path, I suggest sticking with the City Caveman path; it may be a more challenging one, but the view at the top is spectacular.

Day 9. The Caveman Angel vs The Austrian Devil

> *The devil has put a penalty on all things we enjoy in life. Either we suffer in health, or we suffer in soul, or we get fat.*
>
> – Albert Einstein

The devil has arrived.

If I thought the City Caveman Plan was having a giant impact on my lifestyle, well, that is *nothing* in comparison to the momentous event of today – my Austrian girlfriend arrived!

I woke at 4:30am today because my girlfriend, Sonja, is arriving from Vienna. I'm not being a jerk for referring to her as 'the devil,' because she is truly a European beauty, and I am so happy that she has moved here to be with me. So why 'the devil'?

Because she is a little eating and munching devil, and lucky to be so, at 23 years of age with a metabolism that allows her to eat what she wants and when! So, she is the perfect 'devil' partner to inadvertently sabotage my City Caveman Plan. And yes, I know: 34-year-old Mike with 23-year-old Sonja – feel free to bust my chops, but like they say, you are only as old as the girl you wake up next to, right? Yep, lucky me!

Sonja's arrival signifies a giant change in my life. I can no longer make selfish decisions, have numerous weekly piss-ups with the boys, fart as many times as I would like, or leave the flat looking like a Kansas-sized tornado rumbled through. So, while her cheeky eating is a potential challenge for me, I do know that having my loving partner here with me full-time will actually be a positive influence on the arrest of my sloppy, wayward, boozy ways.

Annie, on the other hand, is a little more worried about Sonja's influence, most particularly in terms of the eating plan. I have assured her that I will stay true to the Plan, but only time will tell.

So, a new battle presents itself – the Austrian battle.

When cartoon characters have a decision to make, they have a little angel over one of their shoulders, telling them to do the right thing, and a devil on the other shoulder encouraging the wrong thing. Well, from this day forward, I now have the same thing: on my right lies the Caveman Angel and on the left lies my Austrian Devil!

In the lead up to Sonja leaving her family to come and live in Australia, I did not want to add stress by telling her about my City Caveman Plan. But today when she arrived on another beautiful Sydney day, she said (in that beautiful Austrian accent), 'Ohhhhh Mike, tonight I treat da good dinner for us wit some wine!' It was not the best time to tell her about my City Caveman Plan, but I figured there was no time like the present. The conversation went something like this:

> 'Well, Sonja…ummm, remember that little fitness thing I hinted about a few weeks back?
> 'Yes'
> 'Well, I am eating like a Caveman now.'
> 'What is dis…Caveman?'
> 'Well, I can only eat fresh and healthy foods, and I have daily workouts with no drinks at all for forty days.'
> (Pause, thinking) 'Well, okay. I support you with dis. We try it together, but I still need chocolate.'

And just like that, the City Caveman Plan received the Austrian stamp of approval!

Caveman Tip:

Be honest with friends and family about your City Caveman Plan. Support from loved ones makes the journey a lot more satisfying.

We sorted pretty quickly that I would assume the role of Head Chef Mike, and she would become Clean Freak Head of Cleaning Sonja. This worked for both of us, especially me, given that last time Sonja cooked for me, the Austrian dish she concocted must have had a fat content that extended into three digits! Delicious, but dangerous!

Today was a great day for us, walking around the city, shopping, kissing and (apologies to the prudes) having a cheeky cuddle of course. My Caveman motivation was quite low with all that love on my mind, so cardio day was not going to be easy. This, coupled with my 4:30am start to get to the airport on time, meant I was exhausted toward the end of the day. But Annie would not let me slide any other day, and today was not likely to be an exception. And I was right because, before too long, I received an SMS from Annie that read:

> *Thanks again for lunch on Sunday. Hope you've left the bedroom to train. See you tomorrow at 11:30am.*

Cheeky Annie! Fair point though! Let's just say my cardio training was going to be tough, given that I'd been out of breath for most of the day already.

I took my wobbly legs to the gym and struggled through my 40 minutes of cardio. Abdominal work was really tough today; it is definitely not getting any easier, so I know I still have quite a long way to go. Damn it.

We cooked a brown rice stir fry for dinner. It was fantastic but challenging to watch Sonja have two glasses of wine without me. Of course, a little post-dinner kiss gave me a cheeky little sample of the lingering flavour of the fruity, Kiwi Sauvignon Blanc!

So today I can chalk up a victory for the Caveman Angel. Tomorrow is another battle, and that Austrian Devil will be lurking – but I'm so happy she's here and here to stay!

Annie says: *One thing I will say about Mike – he is truly acting like a caveman. He has gone out, clubbed a young, attractive maiden over the head and dragged her back to his cave for carnal delights! You are getting fully into character aren't you Mikey? Good for you. Companionship and sex is as much a human need as food and water, so I'm glad all his needs are being met. As long as she is going to be supportive, then the more the merrier on the support team!*

Tempting wine and chocolate will be a lot closer now, but unfortunately we cannot lock Mike in solitary confinement for the next thirty-one days. More battles remain, but she will be thanking me for turning her man into one of great strength and endurance!

On a more serious note, partnering up is such a wonderful part of life. Sure, there is a little risk that they end up enjoying some champagne and brie one evening, but so far it sounds like Sonja will be a supportive Caveman partner, and this is fantastic.

Having someone to go for walks with, cook healthy meals with, and have entertaining, non-drinking nights in with can be a perfect complement to the City Caveman Plan. Psychologically for Mike, having a partner move all the way to Australia to be with him can only act as more motivation to improve his life and his health so he can be all he can be in return. And, as Mike struggles with food temptations and challenging workouts, talking about the mental highs and lows of each day with Sonja can only be therapeutic.

So, I will keep my fingers crossed that while the devil lurks, the Caveman Angel and I will keep being victorious for the remaining thirty-one days of our Plan.

Day 10. What's in My Food?

> *Homer: Lisa, would you like a doughnut?*
> *Lisa: No thanks. Do you have any fruit?*
> *Homer: This has purple in it. Purple is a fruit.*
>
> – The Simpsons

It is zero fun cleaning out closets, organising clothes and looking at old bills to determine if you still need to keep them or not. A tooth extraction would have been more fun on this Wednesday evening. Opening the kitchen cupboards is definitely the worst of all the things on my 'to do' list. Single-guy-Mike most likely would have let those items in the cupboard with the 2005 use-by dates sit there until 2008, but with a female in the house, I admit it: I am no longer the boss!

Picture it: rubbish bin overflowing, on a step-ladder and putting my fat head into the cupboard to analyse, clean and throw away things I should have discarded before Sonja arrived.

One item really stuck out; a 'healthy' tomato soup that I obtained some months back.

Last winter I went for a 'run' with my friend Marty. I use that term 'run' lightly; it was more like a 150 metre jog, with about 20 minutes of walking and gossiping about what was planned for the weekend, followed with two minutes of discussion about where we could get 25 or more grams of buttery fat (i.e., a muffin). Anyway, after wishing Marty a good day, I was on my way home when I noticed some pretty promotion girls passing out 'freebie' food. Why wouldn't a guy gravitate towards pretty girls passing out free food? They were giving away 'Sun-Ripened Tomato & Tuscan Herb' powdered soup. The packaging had a waterfall of fresh tomatoes and greens falling into a mug ready to be consumed, making it look like the perfect snack on a cold day. However, if you look at the ingredients you'll see that there's definitely no freshness packed in that powder. A few items that caught my eye were:

Vegetable fat
Malted yeast flavour
Glucose syrup
Stabiliser (470)
Colour
Garlic chilli flavouring
Stabiliser (414)
Stabiliser (340)
Barley malt extract

The question is: what is all this stuff? Is it really food? With a little help from Google, I found that Stabiliser (340) is a food additive called potassium phosphate. It is an *acidity regulator*, *emulsifier* as well as a *stabiliser*[ii]. Am I eating tomato and Tuscan herbs or am I sucking down fake food made by some chemist in a lab? What in the world is this stuff? Where is it made? Why is it in the food? And what does it do to my body? All I know is that cavemen never ate stabilisers, so my fake soup went straight in the bin.

It is a shame that companies are creating 'healthy food mirages' and getting away with it, because the consumer has to look in the fine print to really see the chemical ingredients that are inside.

This information makes me more determined to stick with my City Caveman Plan of fresh food. Like Annie says, if you don't prepare and make it yourself, how can you truly know what's in it?

Caveman Tip:

Stay fresh and healthy in the kitchen, and you will stay fresh and healthy in mind and body.

The leg workout I did with Annie was painful today. However, rather than looking at the weight workouts as a source of discomfort, I am starting to be able to focus on feeling satisfied that I did it, and the buzz the workout provides afterwards. And if I dare even say it, I might be starting to look forward to the next workout right after one ends!

---

ii Food Additive Database, Food Standards Australia New Zealand, February 2007, Copyright Food Standards Australia New Zealand reproduced by permission.

It's Day 10 and while I am still battling every day and still feeling a little sore, I am 25 per cent of the way into my journey. I can go to sleep tonight knowing that I, Mike Jarosky, am still 100 per cent committed to the City Caveman Plan.

Annie says: *We definitely had another great leg session today. I am starting to see definite improvements in Mike's strength and stamina, and the muscles in Mike's legs are even becoming more defined. Over the next two days he should find that he isn't as sore as he was last week, which will not only be a pleasant surprise for him, but it will also make his running more enjoyable.*

As for Mike's big cleanout, the cleaning of his pantry is symbolic of the cleansing he is doing to his body. With his new diet, water and exercise routine, Mike's body is flushing itself of the many toxins he has accumulated over the past few months. All the alcohol, preservatives, colourings, flavourings, thickeners and fat are being peed, poohed or sweated out of him.

And, as he has observed, even foods we assume are healthy due to their labelling or marketing, are actually not as nutritious as we may think. Have a look at any can of goods in the supermarket on your next visit. For example, take a peek at a can of fruit – some have a use-by date that stretches far into the future. For fruit?

Most fresh oranges, kiwis and bananas turn bad in a week's time, yet all the additives and preservatives in the canned varieties magically keep them edible for a month. In my opinion, fresh is best.

At the outset, I did not want to give Mike the technical definition of what he is doing to his body, because it may seem a bit much to take on. But, essentially, he is going through a body detoxification. Of course, rather than tell him this at Day 1 and potentially scare him, I sent him in a bit blind. But, now that he's well on his way, we can boldly say that during his first ten days of change, it is exactly what he has done. He has flushed out the bad chemicals and has learned to replace them with good nutrients, fresh fruit, water and chemical-free food – a simple Caveman Detox!

12

City Caveman Days 11 to 20 – *Battling*

Day 11. Temptation

It is not the great temptations that ruin us; it is the little ones.

– John W. DeForest

Today's workout was not fun. Thursday is officially the killer day, as the first three workout days of the week are fantastic, but they wear me down for my Thursday run.

I really did battle to get through my 40-minute run today. I took a few breaks, had some water, but all in all I made it the full 40 minutes. Abs were a struggle as well, and I wish I had left the gym with my 'gym buzz' but, strangely, I left feeling mad. Why? Well, at the outset I did not want to *go* to the gym in the first place, and then when I arrived I did not want to *be* at the gym, and when I started running I just wanted to be elsewhere. However, I should not bang myself up about it. All days cannot be perfect at the gym and, like everything, even my workouts will have highs and lows.

I know that in the big scheme of things this tired feeling means my workouts are going well. Another little healthy change I have noticed about myself is that *gym tired* is a way better feeling than *hung-over tired*. Going to bed drunk, waking up hung over, sweating like Fat Elvis and spending a full day with that brain-fog feeling of being tired and cranky is certainly no way to live. I definitely enjoy this headspace a lot more.

It has been eleven days now and over the last couple I have, admittedly, become slack with my stretching, which is a *horrible* idea considering I have done a run, leg weights and a run in the last three workout sessions. My mentality has been 'ohhhhhh, just one more set of weights, and then I am done,' and disregarding the fact my stretching sessions are actually the finale of the workout. Big mistake. From here on I must change my mentality and realise that a quick stretch at the beginning, and at least a five-minute stretch at the end, is essential for my body and will make my results arrive faster.

Today was also a day of significant temptation.

Being American, you would think that I would have had my fill of cheeky chicken purchases in my lifetime, especially with my father owning a few KFCs throughout the years. We have spicy Popeye's chicken, KFC, Church's chicken and Boston Market rotisserie chicken. But nothing (and I mean NOTHING) I have ever eaten compares as favourably to the Australian charcoal chicken with stuffing. It simply oozes with flavour, and do not get me started on the flavoursome skin! I could eat the chicken skin for a meal all on its own. The stuffing is usually gone before I can rip one piece off for a meal and, if I eat half a chicken for my dinner, I usually consume the other half before going to bed. I hate to think of how many fat grams are in that!

So here I am. Post-Thursday workout in a sluggish mood, and I pass by the deli section where about twenty barbecue chickens are laid out and looking oh-so good! Temptation right before my eyes. Am I battling? You bet your arse I am.

Caveman Tip:

Temptation is everywhere. Take a deep breath, relax, battle and stay committed to the City Caveman Plan.

And it seemed that temptation just kept rearing its head all day. Sonja and I went for an evening walk and passed by some bars, where we could see and hear people enjoying the drinks that I couldn't have. The City Caveman Plan was starting to sound a little crazy to Sonja. The short version of our chat was that she feels it is a bit too extreme, what with no chocolate, no pizza, no drinks and no deviation whatsoever. She thinks that the City Caveman Plan is making me miss out on some of the things that I truly enjoy. To be honest, I kind of took it to heart that she thinks my personal plan is a little crazy, but I do understand how it might look to her.

My theory is that in extreme circumstances, extreme changes must be made. Look at my eating and drinking of the past – it was shit. And you don't combat shit with just a little less shit; you combat it with a big change – a healthy change. I am at a point where *less* eating and drinking is not good enough. I need a whole new direction and a radical change – and that change, my 180 degree refocusing effort, is the City Caveman Plan.

Isn't it shocking how people who have heart attacks keep eating crap food or go on smoking cigarettes? Or how the famous (and now dead) English soccer player, George Best had a liver transplant due to alcoholism, yet continued drinking afterwards? Well, I am looking at my City Caveman Plan as giving myself a second chance at health and fitness; a second chance at life, actually. And to combat my binge-eating and drinking of the past, I have no choice but to negate it with extreme health and fitness. Will I enjoy some wine and the occasional fish and chips when it is all said and done? Absolutely I will. But for the moment, for right now, I am undergoing a period of change, a period of learning and a period of health.

And to this explanation my Sonja said, 'Okay Mike. Now I understand dis City Caveman Plan.'

***Annie says**: Mike's Thursdays are like being at the bottom of the roller-coaster we keep mentioning. People experience this during the process of undertaking any severe change to the system. If you are breaking one habit and creating a new one, the body initially rejects it because the body is all about keeping the equilibrium, even if that equilibrium is unhealthy. The trick is to realise that there will be down days on the journey, when all you feel like doing is lying on the couch and pigging out, but if you can acknowledge your feelings without giving into them, you will be successful in the end! Persevere! Keep your eye on the prize and dig your heels in when the going gets tough.*

As for the need for a radical change, Mike is absolutely right. There is no point making a half-hearted effort over the forty days, because that would simply be telling your body that you are not serious. Make a severe change to the system, and it will stand to attention and adopt new habits in response. Sure, he will be facing a different challenge regarding training and diet after the forty days of change, but because the process wasn't easy and the results will be so rewarding, I am sure he will not revert back to his old, bad habits.

Sticking to the Plan is also a matter of pride and self-esteem. Mike has made a daily eating and fitness plan. He has told people what he is doing. He faces his Caveman Contract in his bathroom mirror seven nights a week. And he has the end vision of what he wants to look and feel like at the end, so if he cheats or doesn't stick to the plan, his self-esteem will plummet as his subconscious will say to him 'you've lost', 'you can't stick to it', and, 'your pictures at the end are going to look bad now.' People are motivated by seeking pleasure and avoiding pain. Previously, eating junk, being lazy and binge drinking were pleasurable for him. Now, doing those exact same things would cause more psychological pain than the temporary pleasure he would get from indulging – so sticking to the Plan is the better option.

Being lazy and living an unhealthy life is easy, but being active and appreciating your health is the more gratifying route in the end.

Day 12. Oh Shit

Send lawyers, guns and money. The shit has hit the fan.

– Warren Zevon

Friday's writing is really going to stink. Literally. A story from the past…

A few years back in Chicago, I went to my friend Jason's house for the American eating extravaganza of the year, also known as The Super Bowl.

Here is what the Super Bowl means to most Americans:

a a day for food indulgence;
b a day for alcohol indulgence;
c the best TV ads of the year;
d a day for extreme gambling; and
e the championship of American football.

Essentially, in the foreground of most Super Bowl parties is food and booze and, in the background, there is a gridiron game going on. The Super Bowl is one of America's biggest food consumption days, making many a nutritionist weep, but keeping food companies happy as so many Super Bowl fatties keep their businesses thriving.

At Jason's apartment we had an endless combination of margaritas, beer, pizza, spicy buffalo wings, seven-layer Mexican dip, Jason's famous Wisconsin-recipe spicy beef chilli in a bread bowl, and so on. I am sure you get the picture of our Super Bowl Sunday: guys, eating, drinking, sports and farting.

If Super Bowl Sunday is one of happiness and indulgence, Super Bowl Monday is one of hangovers, bloated stomachs and overworked toilets. Well, my Monday was truly a Super, Super Monday.

My girlfriend at the time suggested we go for a Monday morning run. Being that I had to work off Sunday's intake, I thought it would be a good idea. It was a very chilly but nice February morning, and we jogged from my apartment, down to the park and over to Lake Michigan. About 15 minutes into my run, it hit me like a ton of bricks.

'Uh oh.'

'What, do you have a stitch?'

'No. It's my stomach. It's time for my *morning business*, but not enough time to make it to the meeting… if you know what I mean.'

'Oh, you goof! Well, I am going to carry on. I will call you after work.'

'Ugh. Okay, bye.'

Teresa had little sympathy for my situation. Though what could she really do? These sorts of issues are personal, and not even a girlfriend can ease that kind of pain. I was on my own. Due to the coldness and beach closings around the lake, the normal toilets were not available – I had to make a bee-line for my own house. Damn it. Being a few kilometres away from home, I probably ran twice as fast on my way home as I did on the way out, but I just knew it was a race against time to make it into my bathroom!

I was probably about five blocks from my house when… gurgle, grumble, grumble… my stomach was sending me a message: it is time to unload.

All of a sudden, the sharpest of sharp pains rocketed through my insides, bringing my run to a halt and nearly bringing me to my knees. I clinched numerous body parts, praying I would not have an accident right then and there in my neighbourhood. Thankfully at that time of the morning, the streets were empty so no one was around to witness my Super Monday super-pain.

Eventually the pain subsided, so I seized the opportunity to sprint. However, I only made it two blocks further when, *WHAM*, it hit me again. I started to prepare myself mentally for the fact that I was a grown man about to have a childhood accident in the front yard of an apartment block.

At the speed of light, I dropped my pants and before I knew it, had scatter-bombed the front lawn of that building with such force that it almost blew me three steps closer to my apartment. I was probably relieving myself for a good 30 seconds, and I still thank heavens to this day that there were no early-to-work folks coming out of that building at that point in time!

In a long-winded (no pun intended) way, this story is very relevant to a key Caveman change that I experienced in my first two weeks. My time on the toilet has changed; from the hung over-induced hot-wet-fast mode, to firm and floaty – the way it should be.

So these days, as a Caveman there are no more *McShits*, no more brown Jackson Pollock paintings in my toilet bowl, and no more *closing the door, turning the tap and clothes dryer on to hide the explosive noises* when a mate is over. And, even luckier for the masses, my gases have gone from the should-be-bottled-and-used-to-fuel-F16s, to, well, just wind. Everybody wins.

And since we're being so open and frank, I may as well also admit that I've noticed significant changes when tending to the toilet, standing up. With the absence of Coke, Red Bulls, beer and wine, my pee has gone from a dark, stinky yellow, to a clear, good-looking (if that is possible) light yellow stream.

Caveman Tip:

Be conscious of what comes out of your body because it is a tell-tale sign of your inner health.

Okay, I know. That's enough. It is common sense, after all. What I put into my body, must come out. Let's just conclude that the City Caveman Plan is definitely making toilet time a lot more enjoyable.

***Annie says**: Mike's story has put the smile back on my face, which is great because I too had a shitty day today!*

What an unfortunate, but hilarious story. I do pity that lawn and the people who lived in the apartment, especially those on the ground level who might have had their windows open! I also feel sorry for Mike for being in such a painful and awkward predicament, but I am very glad the City Caveman Plan has improved his toilet time so he does not have to embarrass himself in a similar manner here in Australia.

Mike now describes his urine as light yellow, which is exactly the colour he should be aiming for. Whenever you pee, check the colour of your urine and if it is dark yellow or orange, it is a sign that you are not drinking the right amount of water! Drop the soda, drop the processed fruit juice and ease up on the coffee. Making sure you are getting two to three litres of water every day is so important for keeping your body hydrated and healthy!

While the toilet-time subject is a tough one to talk about, it is certainly very, very necessary to monitor. Eating healthy does improve the consistency and smell of faeces – it becomes easier to pass and doesn't stink out the whole house (maybe only the bathroom occasionally). The change in Mike's 'sitting down' time is a fantastic sign that his body is becoming healthier on the inside. Unfortunately, many people workout just for the 'body beautiful' reasons, but we must also respect these important signs, provided by our inner organs.

Day 13. Fitness Fashion

> *Fashion is not something that exists in dresses only. Fashion is in the sky, in the street, fashion has to do with ideas, the way we live, what is happening.*
>
> – Coco Chanel

I will admit to being a *people watcher*. In public places I love observing the way people walk and talk, the way they engage with others, their body language, body shapes and how people dress. I love to watch people and see how they interact in their world; and at the gym, it's no different.

However, over the last couple of weeks the joy of observation has left me bewildered by some pretty alarming fitness fashions. I mean, how is that a highly paid, sharply dressed banker can enter the gym in such impressive apparel, but then emerge from the locker room wearing dirty, purple sweatpants and black socks? What's going on there?

So, for Day 13 I think a little fashion advice is called for; after all, the clothes maketh the man (and woman), right? And if we think we look good, then we will also start to feel good!

For the men:

a Shirts – It's great that you saw AC/DC in Wagga Wagga back in '87 but, unlike wine, shirts do not necessarily age well. Box those 20-year-old shirts up and sell them on eBay; or better still, burn them! Whatever you do, don't wear them to the gym!

b Shorts – Spandex or lycra shorts are great…as *undershorts*. Yes, they provide us with great support and keep *our boys* from bouncing all over the place, but, on their own, spandex and lycra are tacky (unless you're an Olympic sprinter where showcasing the front-bump is a necessary part of the intimidation process). So, let's make the gym a happier place and cover up those lycra shorts with some proper sports shorts.

c Hair – Now I'm not talking about a mullet hairstyle (although that, too, can be quite offensive at times); I'm talking about *body* hair. If you sport a hairy back, please reconsider wearing a singlet; or if you must, could you please wax or shave beforehand? You may not be aware but your sweat can get all caught up in the masses of follicles, which creates your own personal Niagara Falls every time you move about in the gym. So for everyone's sake, please cover up that body hair with some appropriate attire.

And so what of the girls in the gym? I think due to the sheer volume of beauty and fashion magazines out there, women seem to have fewer gym-fashion faux-pas than the guys do, but here are a couple of my pet peeves when it comes to women's fashion:

a Muffin Top – I am definitely carrying my chub, but I do give some effort to try and cover it up with the right type of shirt. Unfortunately, some females haven't quite understood that message and are still attempting to squeeze themselves into Paris Hilton-sized fitness gear. But ladies, I need to be the bearer of bad news: when you slouch over the bike, it is all rolling together and overhanging, and it is not doing you any favours. Please try and find appropriate shirts that fit your body type.

b Exposed undies – Whether you know it or not, most heterosexual men possess a kind of a sixth sense when it comes to nudity. What this means is, if we can sense that some flesh, or something flesh-related, is available for the looking, then we'll do our darndest to take a good, hard, long look. So, if you are wearing an outfit that exposes your underwear, make no mistake that we will stare at you/it. The best way I can describe it is that it's like a reflex or an instinct; we simply have no control over it. So, if you do not wish to attract mindless staring, then please wear some gear that covers up *your gear* when you workout.

I think if we could all heed some simple fashion tips like these, the gym world could be a much happier place for everyone!

Come to think of it, what we wear can impact on our progress and performance quite significantly. Think about it. Rugby players come to the stadium in their street clothes, change into their uniforms and come out of the tunnel with a whole new mentality that readies them to do battle on the field. And my City Caveman Plan is the same; I change into my gym gear, switch into my Game Day mentality, and I'm ready to continue battling within my health and fitness journey. Did my fashionable workout gear make me stronger or faster today? No. But it *did* help me get into the mental space I needed in order to get my health and fitness back on track.

Caveman Tip:

Become the part by dressing the part. It will help you get into your Game Day mentality every day.

Annie says: *I think the most important fashion-related issue in the gym is the support and comfort that your shoes provide you with. Old shoes can damage your feet, ankles and knees, which can then cause problems with your back and upper body as well. Poor shoes can also cause you to slip during training, so buying the right pair of shoes is definitely fitness fashion tip number one in my book! Try not to worry too much about the colours of your shoes or how they look with the rest of your outfit; the priority should be that your arch is properly placed, that your pronation or supination (the direction your feet roll out or in when you walk/run) is adequately supported, and that you have the comfort you need to perform the City Caveman workouts effectively and comfortably.*

And, while at first I thought Mike was displaying a splash of snobbiness with his fashion writing, I couldn't agree more with his point about getting into the Game Day mentality. We dress for the occasion, and we should, therefore, dress appropriately for our Caveman workouts. That doesn't mean we need to spend $1,500 on a full-body swim-skin that the Olympians wear, but it does mean taking enough pride in our appearance to help develop and maintain your Game Day approach in the gym.

Of course, when you have completed your forty days as a City Caveman and have a slimmer, sexier body, it's not only the fashion in the gym that you will be thinking about; you will also find yourself with new and exciting fashion opportunities for every occasion and situation!

Day 14. The Price of Good Health

> *It takes only one drink to get me drunk. The trouble is, I can't remember if it's the thirteenth or the fourteenth.*
>
> – George Burns

I felt like my body had earned the Sunday recovery day this week, so Sonja and I went for a beautiful walk in the 22 degree weather, followed by lunch on the beach where Annie and some of her mates joined us. Like Annie, her friends were also in the fitness industry, yet everybody at the table was eating fried goodies, right there in front of me! Oh, the temptation!

Last night we went to a birthday party in the city and, of course, it was a dry party for me. I ran into a few friends who I had not seen in a few weeks, and it was interesting to hear their responses when I told them I was off the drinks for a few weeks:

> 'Really? Did drinking become a problem for you?'
> 'Oh, come on, and don't be a wuss, go get yourself a drink!
> 'Come on mate, three drinks won't kill you.'

It was pretty humorous and all in good spirits, but I will admit it's still tough to be socialising sober. But I am proud of the fact that I have made it this far.

Another thought crossed my mind regarding the fact it's now been two weeks of no drinking: alcohol savings. Drinking is bloody expensive in a major city, so, I thought, why not do the calculations? And so I did.

Earlier on, I detailed my weekly eating and drinking, so I decided to work out how much money the City Caveman Plan has saved me. I took those consumption statistics, computed an average price per drink, taking into consideration whether the drink was consumed at the bars or at home (cheaper), and the math flowed from there. And this is what I found:

Chubby Mike's Drinking			
Amount	**Type**	**$**	**Total**
2	Glasses of Red Wine	$5	$10
2	Coronas	$3	$6
1	Bottle of White Wine	$28	$28
7	Schooners of James Squires	$6	$42
6	Glasses of White Wine	$8	$48
1	Vodka Martini	$15	$15
2	Rum & Cokes	$7	$14
2	Tequila Shots	$8	$16
2	Bottles Red Wine	$30	$60
	Total		**$239**
	52 weeks per year		**$12,428**

Can you believe that? $239 per week spent on alcohol. Yikes. And the news gets worse because when I calculate $239 x 52 weeks, it reveals a staggering $12,428 wasted per year on booze. Of course, the good news is that in the past two weeks I have saved nearly $480. And let me tell you, I have noticed myself going to the automatic teller machines a lot less too. I have noticed constantly having $50 notes in my pocket, rather than spending them frivolously on bottles of wine during the week.

Analysing the financial impact of the alcohol consumption led me to think about the other effects it had on my life. I asked myself a few simple questions:

Does alcohol make me feel good? **Yes** (in the very short term)
Is it good for my body? **No**
Do I get good drunk-sleep? **No**
Is it good for my mind? **No**
Is it cheap? **No**
Am I in a good mood after a night's drinking session? **No**
Can I have good workouts hung-over? **No**
Do I eat well while drunk/hung-over? **No**

Wow. So why did I drink so much? It takes some time to really analyse yourself and determine 'I am a drinker.' A few times in my past I had given thought to whether I could really stop, but until now, I never actually tried. At this stage, when this Plan is completed, I am thinking I will turn my 'habitual' drinking into 'celebratory drinking' on fewer occasions.

So, with two of six Caveman weeks now gone by, this means I am officially 33 per cent of the way there. An important milestone? Yes, I think so, because over the past few days, I have noticed that *doubt* is increasingly being replaced by a Caveman confidence. Ohhhhh, I am still aware that change and completing the City Caveman Plan won't be easy – there will still be ups and downs and cravings that continue to come and go – but, rather than feeling 'I am not sure if I can do it', I think I have turned a corner where I feel like *I can do it*.

Caveman Tip:

Dedication will replace doubt with feelings of 'I *am* doing it, I will *continue* to do it and I *know* I can do it.'

Doubt is out, and an extra $239 per week is in! So, the City Caveman Plan is not only enhancing my health but it's also improving my finances! At the end of week two, it's looking good.

Annie says: *Today certainly was a lovely meal in Watson's Bay with Mike, Sonja and some other friends – beachside food and wine with spectacular harbour views.*

I felt a bit guilty eating chips in front of Mike, but Sunday is my self-awarded 'cheat day', which he can think about introducing at the end of his forty days. It is pretty self-explanatory: after the forty days of change, if you are eating well during the week, you might reward yourself on Sunday by eating whatever you want. By having your own 'Sunday cheat day', it is easier to stop the food cravings during the week because you can look forward to your deviance day! Plus, it ensures you don't feel like you are completely missing out on some of life's cheeky culinary delights. This way, eating a little junk food becomes a treat, rather than something to feel guilty about.

It's great that Mike is realising that by not drinking he is not only saving his liver, but his money too. Aside from containing empty calories, alcohol is very expensive, which is one of the reasons I hardly ever drink. I also hate feeling hung over. And, being a control freak (I hear Mike agreeing!), I also hate that feeling of being out of control, which can happen if you overindulge.

I am also a firm believer that you can have a good time without getting drunk. If you disagree, maybe it is time you look at your own reasons for drinking alcohol. I remember going to many a party and people assuming I was taking party drugs because of my high energy levels. I wasn't corny enough to tell them I was high on life, but the truth is that for me, like a good workout, dancing makes me feel high, and when you're fit you can dance all night without the assistance of any synthetic substances.

I would encourage you to work out how much you're saving on the City Caveman Plan and record how you feel when you socialise without alcohol. To begin with, you're bound to feel a little left out or conspicuous, but I guarantee you will be pleasantly surprised with your next day's energy and your ability to enjoy more of life's experiences with a chemical-free mind and body.

Day 15. Understanding Change

Things do not change. We change.

– Henry David Thoreau

I think I finally get it.

Before detailing what it is that I actually *get*, I will share a weird quirk (yes, another one) about myself. Unbeknownst to me, for some odd reason I tend to do my best thinking in three places: the shower, on the treadmill, or sitting on the toilet when no reading material is available.

Today, my epiphany arrived while I was in the gym shower. I think I finally realised why my previous efforts to live a healthy life always came up short.

A nifty chart to explain is below…

Figure 1

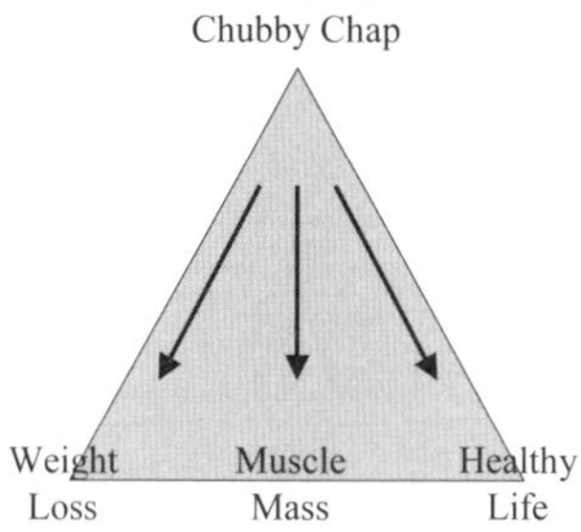

I am the chubby chap at the top of the chart. I want all three of the elements at the bottom of the chart: fat loss, muscle mass and a healthy life. However, in the past when I went to the gym, I've had no workout plan, and at home I've had no eating plan. Therefore, I've had no real means to achieve the third component on the pyramid either; yet I know that I want to.

That has been me in a nutshell.

Prior to my City Caveman Plan, I have been battling the challenge to create a healthy life for a few years now.

My pattern was to head for the 'I want it now' cheating cure of vitamin/fat loss pills, thinking these will be my saviour. Very wrong. What was missing? The element of *change*; rather than changing my lifestyle of fatty foods and too much alcohol, I was looking for the easy cure, and if there's one place where shortcuts won't work, it's my body.

So what is it that I now know, that I didn't realise before?

I now understand that the only thing standing between me and the fat loss, toned body and healthier life that I desire, is *change*.

This means making a fitness plan, understanding proper diet and going without all the pleasure consumption I was indulging in. I wanted the physical change, yet I never began the process of the mental change. The process of how I *should* have been thinking is below.

Figure 2

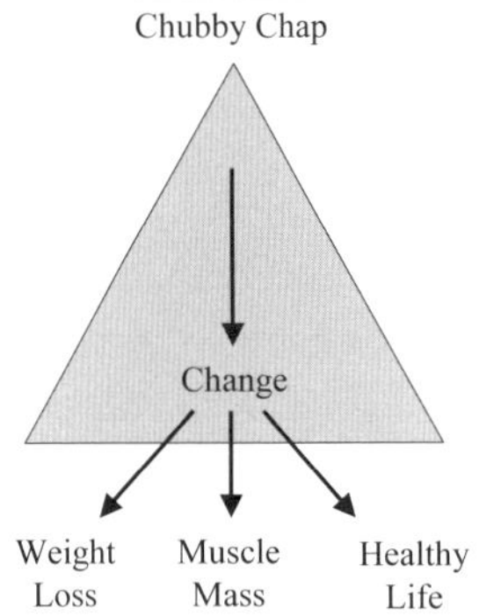

It is so clear to me now that to obtain fat loss and muscle mass and lead a healthier life, I must *change* first! A tennis player who wants to play professional golf cannot just sign up for a tournament and expect to play. He must understand the process of change (learning a new swing, golf rules, etc.) required to become something he is currently not; and my fitness progression is the same. I now understand that within the process of change:

a the binge drinking nights are not on,

b the late night Macca's runs are over,

c daily battles occur each day that I have to take head-on,

d cravings will come and go and come again,
e there is temptation from mates to deviate from the City Caveman Plan,
f battling through soreness is a rough part of the journey, and
g there will be good days, and there will be bad days.

Caveman Tip:

Focus 100 per cent of your efforts to *change*, and the physical rewards will soon be yours.

I am certainly no sports psychologist, but for me, this idea makes sense. And by gaining a better understanding of myself like this, I think achieving change through the City Caveman Plan is going to be a whole lot more interesting and fun.

***Annie's say**: Nice little triangles Mike! Change is often a scary word for a lot of people because, unfortunately, we all tend to prefer to be in our comfort zones. Coming from a family who tended to move every four years, I know first-hand that change can be scary and is stressful at first, but it can also be very exciting and an effective way for us to improve ourselves and become stronger. Life is like a treadmill; you have to keep walking because if you stand still, you will go backwards. Not being willing to change is the equivalent of standing still because life will change around us. Of course, you need to regularly stop and ask yourself whether you are changing for the better or for the worse.*

Mike does 'get it'. He understands that becoming healthy is like cooking a meal – you cannot just say 'I want risotto.' You must understand all the ingredients, the cooking methods and the timing required to make that meal. Wanting something without having a plan or strategy to achieve the change will see you on a path to nowhere.

A lot of people know what it takes to be healthy or lose weight, but there is a big difference between knowing it consciously and writing a daily plan to put it into effect. And that is where Mike is currently positioned.

In order to bring change into your world and create the healthy life you desire, print out the City Caveman Plan of what you will eat and the exercises you will do, stick it on your fridge or bathroom mirror, and tick them off after you have done them. And do it every day! This will give you a sense of direction and accomplishment. And this daily change will translate into a life change that will see you feeling and looking your best.

Create your own conscious path of where you want to go, and you will achieve your personal goals.

Day 16. Face-a-tarian

> *The second day of a diet is always easier than the first. By the second day, you're off it.*
>
> – Jackie Gleason

I chat with my neighbour once in a while, who I also see at the gym on occasion. I don't know her too well, but she scoffs at any sort of City Caveman Plan, as her UK blood would never allow her to give up drinking four to five nights a week!

Today she told me how insane her flatmate is, because she is already at a size next-to-nothing, yet she has just started *the* low-carb diet to lose five more kilograms.

We discussed how crazy that diet is. Seriously – a diet that disallows the consumption of fruit? How could anyone put themselves through this? I asked my UK mate if she thought she could do that diet, but she said 'no', because she doesn't eat meat. I had forgotten as previously she had informed me that she was, in fact, a *faceatarian*.

Yes, you read that correctly. A face-a-tarian.

This was certainly a new word to me. The definition of a faceatarian is actually the *converse* of the other words with '-atarian' suffixes. For example, a vegetarian eats veggies, but she explained that some vegetarians eat fish or chicken and she wanted to distinguish herself from them. A faceataraian, therefore, is one who will not eat anything that has a face.

I wasn't sure if I should have started laughing or just called her bizarre and wished her a fine day.

Missing out on a nicely grilled steak, not being able to have grilled prawns on Christmas, or never having a Sunday fish-and-chips after a sunny, 28-degree day at the beach? I would not fare well if I signed up for a life like that! Similarly, I remember hearing an American doctor on the Aussie radio talking about healthy diet, and he was endorsing an eating plan that consisted only of vegetables and plants, claiming that we can obtain all of the required nutrients from a plant-only diet.

Denying myself the pleasures of tasty food is out of the question in my book. You can't adopt a healthy lifestyle if you are living with such restrictions.

Taking on this City Caveman Plan has definitely taught me that healthy can still be tasty. Take tonight for example. Using a chicken breast I had in the fridge, I took some fat-free lemon yoghurt, dropped it into the blender and added a bit of paprika, Cajun herbs, ground black pepper and garlic. I then spread the spicy and sweet lemon sauce over the chicken, and I put it on the grill for five minutes. That lemon spiced chicken breast, on top of a rocket, tomato, cucumber, red pepper and mushroom salad was absolutely fantastic! Bollocks to you faceatarians!

I sure do miss a bit of junk food in my eating plan; however, not once during my first three weeks have I felt like I've gone without. Not once have I been hungry, and not once would I ever consider one of these fad-diets as an alternative method to achieve my goals.

My Caveman way of eating less than 10 fat grams per meal has tested my creativity in the kitchen, which has been challenging, but it is certainly better than limiting your diet to items without a face! I believe that wacky eating trends are unsustainable for the long term and, therefore, equate to zero fun.

Caveman Tip:

Ignore bullshit diet trends and keep your Caveman cooking simple. Keep it fresh and get creative – it can still be fun and full of taste.

Okay, on a less odd note, my run today was a mixed bag. Tuesday is proving to be my easiest day (though still not painless), as I tend to feel quite fresh, it being so early in the week and all. I guess I should try and relish my Tuesday 'bounce' on the treadmill because Wednesday's leg workout with Annie usually leaves me with a flat tyre for my Thursday run! But, that aside, I think I do feel lighter on the treadmill and better in my jeans, so without getting on the scale or taking fatty-photos again, I am confident that I am making progress with my simple, yet efficient workouts. I am thankful that in designing the Workout Plan, Annie stayed true to my demand of not undertaking any ridiculous looking exercises in the gym, which might draw attention to me.

So, off to bed for this tired chap. Right before I shut the computer down, on comes a burger commercial. Ugh. Cravings, cravings, go away…

Annie says: *Okay, well the faceatarian thing might be a little extreme, but having been raised a vegetarian myself, I have to tell you – it's not so bad!*

I agree that nothing beats a roast dinner with real meat, but the idea that vegetarians eat nothing but brussels sprouts is a misconception. Most veggie meals are low in fat and chemical-free. But free of taste? Certainly not!

Regardless of what side of the fence you sit on, the point is that you have to choose what is comfortable for your lifestyle, and it is then up to you to make it nutritional and tasty!

I used to compete in fitness competitions, which meant I had to go on special diets, and I have to tell you – I hated every second of it. I would rather exercise like a madman, rather than have to diet so strictly again. My philosophy these days is 'everything in moderation.' I do not deny myself any food and my diet is mostly vegetarian due to habit and ease of cooking, but it is never what you'd call strict or prohibitive.

It is no surprise that junk food is so popular, with every second commercial being for something high in fat, sugar and calories. However, there is a difference between just seeing those commercials and acting upon them. I'm pleased to say that Mike is definitely in a significant period of change, so rest assured that those cravings and temptations will soon prove to be less appealing with time.

Be patient, Mike. The tide is turning your way.

Day 17. Fight, Squeeze and Shape

> *The more you sweat in training, the less you bleed in battle.*
>
> – Sun Tzu

Today, Annie's son is not feeling well, so we won't be doing a legs workout together. I should be feeling happy to be able to train at my own pace, right? Wrong. I actually prefer my workout sessions with her because while they are tough, they are also efficient and, in the end, very rewarding. It is a true mental break when she tells me what exercise is next, how many sets and reps need to be done, and she motivates me when she sees me slowing down. She says 'jump', and I don't need to think about it; I just ask 'how high?'

So, without Annie, my enthusiasm to complete my solo leg workout was pretty low. But I had a new source of motivation to tap into: verbal spats with Sonja.

Sonja has been having a rough time being in a new country, with new people, new live-in boyfriend, new apartment, new everything! And this morning the stress culminated in our first big fight.

The beauty and uniqueness of our relationship lies in our opposite personalities. I am quite laid-back, while Sonja is the fiery one. So, we usually meet somewhere in the middle and get along just fine. However, when we do have a row, this difference can often result in an argument that becomes quite heated. And this morning was one of those times, only worse.

Now I don't mind confrontation, but I am more prone to taking deep breaths and quietly excusing myself from the situation in order to regain my thoughts and have a civil, less explosive conversation later.

So that's what I did, and I headed to the gym. Of course, I arrived annoyed and fired up, but quickly zoned out during my 20-minute run. Game Day mentality wasn't required since anger gave me all the motivation I needed for the workout.

My legs workout was intense. I felt so angry; not so much at Sonja anymore, I was just in a shit, shit mood, and so I took it out on the weights. For the first time, I actually looked forward to tomorrow's fatigue.

I still felt angry when I reached my abs workout. And it helped me find a new technique: *the abdominal squeeze*.

During my first two weeks, I had been getting some good abs workouts, but today I took it to a whole new level. Rather than just going through the rocking-up-and-down motions of crunches and side sit-ups, etc, when I reached the top of the sit-up position, I gave a tight 'squeeze' of my ab muscles. It immediately increased the intensity of the training.

When my brother had given me his abdominal program, Annie had told me to be mindful of not going through the motions without thinking about the movement during the ab exercises. She told me to 'squeeze' at the top of every sit-up, side sit-up, or any exercise I did that involved my abs.

Unfortunately, it has taken me two weeks to actually *squeeze*, but I finally did, and wow! It's such a different workout. Of course, I did have to delay the squeeze a few times, in order to avoid Mother Nature taking over and letting rip with one of those clear-the-room type farts!

Caveman Tip:

During resistance exercises…focus, concentrate and *squeeze*. It will increase the intensity of your exercise.

A full workout, a bit of exhaustion and a nice walk home seemed to temper my angry mood to the point where I was feeling better by the time I arrived home. After a quick shower I caught a glimpse of myself in the full-length mirror. My thoughts? Disappointment? Actually no. Not the same disappointment as when I took those disastrous photos just one week into the Plan. I can notice some small changes in my body; my jeans are fitting more loosely, and I am even tightening a notch on my belt buckle. In fact, when I saw my neighbour the other day, she said I looked 'tanned and well'. That was nice, but *I* am not seeing any major changes yet. Still. Unfortunately.

I know that I definitely started this City Caveman Plan with a body shaped like a pear; and now? Well, I still feel like that pear, but perhaps a few kilograms lighter. My weight has fallen, but my shape remains a *pear*!

Oh well, there is nothing more that I can do except trust that the Plan will eventually do its thing and whip my body into the shape I want it to be. And also, I am willing to consider the fact that it may well be my own inability to see the changes. I mean, maybe, when I look at myself, I am so used to seeing my reflection in a certain way that I am blind to the changes.

Despite the fights, squeezing and shape blindness, temptation still persists. Sonja's 'welcome to Australia' Tim Tam balls that I bought last week were still sitting right next to my bottled water, still unfinished and still calling my name every time I looked at them! In fact, there was a moment when they called so loudly that I actually stuck my hand in that bag, grabbed two of those chocolate-covered treats and started twirling those little balls of joy in my hand. Until, with slight hesitation, I put them back in the bag. I know. Not good – on many levels! That delicious chocolate taste would have been so amazing on this topsy-turvy Wednesday; but this Caveman will be good and continue to stick to the Plan.

Wow, what a Wednesday. A glass of Hunter Valley red would be golden right now but instead I shall savour the apology, kiss and freshly grilled tuna-steak and veggies that Sonja has prepared for me. It's great to have that little devil back in the good books again!

Annie says: *First off, an apology to Mike for missing the workout today. I love training legs, so missing out was sad for me, but this mum must look after her little fella. I am sorry to hear he had a fight with the missus, but letting your anger out in the weights room is always a great way to let it go.*

Actually, that is one thing I advise my psychology clients: it's absolutely okay to feel angry; in fact, it's human. But what is not okay is to get into an argument with someone and stay there until it escalates into something really mean and nasty.

If arguments become heated or start to get personal or reach a fever pitch with an eight-out-of-ten intensity level, then leave. Temporarily, I mean. Just walk away, think about it, cool down, let some steam off with a run or some weights training, and then go back and talk about it calmly and rationally. This way you have more chance of communicating effectively and resolving the conflict.

What Mike describes, about not seeing the changes that others notice, is quite a common occurrence. The fact is, we see and scrutinise ourselves every single day, so the physical changes that are very subtle and gradual may not be as visible to us as they are for those who see us less frequently. And, as we've already mentioned, our internal changes do not necessarily follow the same rate of change as our external changes. For example, I had a client who was a slim man, though he had once been obese, and he told me that he still 'felt' like a fat guy. This happens because our self-esteem can take a while to catch up to our outer metamorphosis. And that's exactly why changing the inner psyche is equally as important.

Now as for those chocolate balls – well done on putting them down, Mike! This is another fantastic sign that you are battling and winning! So many people 'comfort eat' to seek an instant but false psychological comfort after a challenging day, just like you had. But you did it! You won another battle.

Congratulations, Mike. Maybe just try to keep your battling limited to the City Caveman Plan instead! That way, you could save your relationship AND your health!

Day 18. Healthy Drugs & Acclimatising the Body

> *A man's health can be judged by which he takes two at a time: pills or stairs.*
>
> – Joan Welsh

'What is dry bark?'
'Ummm, I'm not really sure, but it really works.'
'Okay.'

One is forgiven for thinking this could be a conversation with the landscaper who visited my house today. But since I live on the 11th floor of an apartment building and don't have a lawn to tend to, it wasn't.

Out of curiosity, prior to my Thursday run I went into the vitamin store to suss out some of the products they sell.

I was approached by a friendly, fit, young girl who kindly asked me if I needed help. I told her I was almost three weeks into a workout plan, and I was wondering what I could use to help me in my fitness pursuit. She brought four products around:

Weight management pills, four pills daily (~ $110)
Creatine, powder (~ $90)
Stamina enhancer, three pills daily (~ $90)
Multivitamin, two pills daily (~ $40)

She told me the whole lot would serve me well for a month's time. She said that the weight management pills would speed up my metabolism, the creatine would make me grow bigger, the stamina enhancer would increase my energy and the multivitamin was to make sure I got all the vitamins in my system I might not be getting via my food intake.

I had no idea about the actual contents of these 'vitamins', so I took a peek at one of the bottles and noticed 'dry bark' was one of the ingredients. Dry bark?

Intrigued by all the chemistry, I couldn't help but comment. 'Bloody hell, you must be a doctor to prescribe all this stuff.' To which, she replied, 'No, no, but trust me, it's all good.'

It's all good? $230 worth of pills is all good? Dry bark is all good? Swallowing nine pills and a powder concoction every day is all good?

It wasn't that long ago when Ephedra was banned in the United States. The vitamin companies were selling it like hotcakes, and it wasn't until a professional baseball player died as a result of the drug that the government recognised Ephedra was, essentially, an over-the-counter narcotic.

These outlets rake in billions of dollars in revenue every year, yet these so-called 'vitamin' companies are essentially selling drugs in an unregulated industry, with no medical involvement, even when some of their items have resulted in consumer deaths!

That's all I needed to know to make my decision.

I will stick with my City Caveman Plan, which means no 'it's all good' pills or powders for me! *I* am going to make sure that *I* know what *I* am putting into *my* body.

So today, not only did I save my $50 that would usually have been invested into some Thursday night booze, but I also saved another $230 by walking out of that 'vitamin' store.

Caveman Tip:

Stop trusting corporations with your health. Put your faith and trust in healthy, fresh Caveman foods and efficient Caveman exercises.

Last night I had a chat with a friend of mine. She is part of the regular drinking group, currently fighting her own fitness battle, but cheeky dinners and way too many drinks are still part of her weekly lifestyle. We just had the normal gossip-chat, and she asked me what I was up to for the weekend. I said there were a few things on, but I was still not drinking. When she asked me, 'For how long?' I told her 'Forty days.'

She then said, 'Shit, I could never do that.'

Which got me thinking about sacrifice.

Coming up to my 35th birthday, I will have been alive around 13,000 days! That's a big number, isn't it? So, out of 13,000 days, how much of a sacrifice is 40 of them? It's about 0.3 per cent, to be exact; which is pretty close to zero. A pretty minuscule investment of time to achieve long-term good health, right?

I am just re-reading that last thought, and there is too much of a negative connotation for my liking. *Sacrifice* should not be used in that sentence. I *should* be saying how great it is to make a 40-day change that will improve the health of my remaining 18,000+ days of living!

I'm almost three weeks in, and I still need to work on changing my mindset. My Plan is no longer about *sacrificing* my binge drinking and eating days; it's about *embracing* a new life and lifestyle that will leave me feeling better mentally, looking better physically and enjoying myself in the future.

Another semi-milestone was reached today. I am no longer feeling sore from my workouts. I am still pushing hard, but instead of that body-shock soreness, I think I'm actually getting fit. It's kind of like climbing Mount Everest (which I've been watching on the Discovery Channel). People who climb the world's tallest mountain do not arrive at the bottom and then step on the gas pedal and head straight for the top, at warp speed. Instead, they spend numerous weeks acclimatising to the altitude and the environment. They hike up to where it's challenging, then stop. There they'll camp until they get accustomed to the atmosphere, and then they continue further up the summit. A mountaineer knows that to be successful they must travel slowly, listen to their body and follow what it tells them.

And I think I'm learning to do the same. My body has been subjected to three weeks of leg weights, jumping rope, chest exercises, long runs and great ab workouts, for the first time ever. And slowly, but surely, it is becoming accustomed to the physicality of it all. Don't get me wrong though; the soreness has gone, but I am still tired from my workouts. However, instead of muscle pain, a good sleep and a nice stretch to warm up is the only cure I seem to need these days.

Okay, it's 10pm on a Thursday. My computer is on my lap, and the Austrian Devil is on the couch. Time to make a swap.

Annie says: *The supplement debate! I am not totally against supplements and multivitamin tablets. However, I only believe in taking supplements in educated, moderate doses. Did you notice how I said 'educated'? I say that because I am a little disheartened by the girl who helped Mike out with his month full of supplements. She does not know Mike, she does not know Mike's body or his history and, therefore, she should not be telling Mike what to buy because she is not making an educated assessment of Mike's needs.*

I took a multivitamin tablet while I was pregnant, and I take one now for breastfeeding. I spoke about this with my doctor, and he said it was okay by him. Unfortunately, not many people even consider discussing their supplement intake with their doctor and, therefore, they are unaware of the risks and potential harm these pills could do to their body. I am not sure what was in the weight management pills or stamina enhancer, so I cannot professionally comment on them. However, all supplements should be taken as a complement to a healthy diet, rather than in place of one. This is so important to understand. Since the City Caveman Eating Plan is so low in fat and so full of natural sources of vitamins and minerals, I can confidently say that Mike does not need to spend a single dollar on synthetic vitamins or minerals, let alone hundreds of dollars! Funnily enough, 'dry bark' actually does sound like something a caveman would eat, but I think we can give it a miss and just stick to our 'au naturel' Eating Plan.

It's also great to see Mike changing his mindset and acclimatising to his new lifestyle. Mike's mind is getting used to motivating him to workout, and his body is getting accustomed to the daily workouts. Mike is also right in that what he is doing is not 'bad', nor is he 'sacrificing' something he should keep hold of. Instead, he is becoming healthy, positive, richer and happy!

And as for Mike's muscles becoming used to the workouts and not being as sore as he used to be. This is good on one hand, because it means he is learning how to cope with the loads we are placing on him; yet, on the other hand, it says to me that he may need to be challenged in new ways. So, Mike, brace yourself. I am going to throw a curveball at your legs in the near future, and I look forward to seeing how you cope! And yes, Mike, being a sadist Caveman advisor and a fitness professional do go hand-in-hand!

Day 19. The Austrian Devil Cooks

> *My wife is the worst cook in the world. At my house, we pray after we eat.*
>
> – Rodney Dangerfield

I came home from a hard workout today to be greeted by Sonja, who said, 'Michael, I am going to do da cooking tonight.'

Ohhhhhh shit. The City Caveman Eating Plan is in trouble.

She told me she was going to make a winter chilli. All I could visualise was the butter, fattening meat, cheese and sour cream she was likely to use in her recipe. Oh dear. The Austrian Devil was out to play.

'Sonja, please, please, we have to make it low-fat or I will have to find something else to eat. Annie would severely injure me if I had a fatty meal for dinner.'

'Ohhhhh, come on, Mike. Just dis one night I cook for you. One night won't be bad for you.'

'Sonja, pleeeeeeeeease, no. How about I look on the internet for some low-fat recipes?'

From Sonja, I hear a huge *sigh* coupled with that *look*, which she fires right at me like an arrow on a mission.

I know this has been hard for Sonja. She arrives in her new home on the other side of the world, and she cannot even have a pizza and a glass of wine with her boyfriend because he claims to be living like a caveman. I do feel for her and, yes, my Caveman endeavour is somewhat selfish; but, when you are worse for wear health-wise, a selfish decision to make a change is not a negative thing. In a way I'm doing it for her, for us, because being healthy ensures I have a future!

Caveman Tip:

It's your life, and it's your health – it's okay to be selfish about it…because your well-being, your health and ultimately your happiness will positively affect your loved ones.

So, while Sonja did the chopping and preparation, I did the online research. I was determined to find a low-fat version of that chilli but, unfortunately, I couldn't. So, we kind of played it by ear, making it up as we went along, and, I must say, it turned out to be one of the tastiest chillies I have ever had! Garlic, tomatoes, chicken, spice, onion and more! Full credit goes to Sonja for a fantastically yummy chilli, which was stripped of all the naughty ingredients. See? That just goes to show: with a little effort and a bit of creativity, you can take what would have been a full-fat meal and turn it into a healthy, tasty dinner.

While we were eating our chilli, an advertistment came on the television for some abdominal exercise machine. What a load of crap! 'Lose inches while watching TV' it promised, as they showed an elderly woman doing sit-ups in front of the television. Lose inches? From one exercise? Who are these people kidding? The commercial continues, 'It folds under your bed for easy storage.' Between you and me, I reckon if it can slide so easily under your bed, then it can also slide right out into the driveway, to be picked up with the rest of the trash!

After checking the nightly, online sports news, I took a look at the national news headlines, and being a fan of the occasional gamble, the first headline I noticed on MSNBC.com was: *Las Vegas Tourists Taken for a Ride on the Strip*[iii]. Curious, I clicked on the link, and I could not believe my eyes when I read the following:

---

iii May 2007, 'Las Vegas tourists taken for a ride on the Strip', <http://www.msnbc.msn.com/id/18849135/>, Used with permission of The Associated Press © 2008 All Rights Reserved.

> *There's lazy, and then there's Las Vegas lazy.*
>
> *In increasing numbers, Las Vegas tourists exhausted by the four miles of gluttony laid out before them are getting around on electric 'mobility scooters'. Forking over about $40 a day and their pride, perfectly healthy tourists are cruising around Las Vegas casinos in transportation intended for the infirm.*
>
> *'It was all the walking,' 27-year-old Simon Lezama said on his red Merits Pioneer 3. Lezama, a trim and fit-looking restaurant manager from Odessa, Texas, rented it on Day 3 of his five-day vacation, 'and now I can drink and drive, be responsible and save my feet.'*

I wasn't sure whether to start laughing or crying. What a sad state our culture is in when individuals are so lazy that they would rather use transportation for people with disabilities than their own feet. I wonder if Simon Lezama also wears an elderly diaper so he can crap in his pants without wasting time in the toilets? Only in America!

Well, I declined the mobility scooter option and walked to the gym earlier today. My chest and back workout turned out to be a gruelling one. I couldn't find that fancy abdominal machine, so I did some extra sit-ups the old fashioned way, using my newfound *squeeze* method, and promptly left the gym feeling like I'd done a damn good City Caveman workout.

Annie's say: *I am glad Mike did not succumb to a fatty chilli and that he and Sonja managed to find a tasty, low-fat option. When you're willing to be creative in the kitchen, it isn't too hard to enjoy a tasty and low fat eating plan. The internet gives us access to a whole new world of recipes, so you can find all sorts of options when looking for nutritious and tasty meals.*

Now, as for calling the City Caveman Plan selfish, this is true to a certain extent, but as he mentioned, it's not totally selfish because Sonja will also benefit in the long run.

You have to remember that when you achieve a new level of health, you will have more energy and you won't be so grumpy or hung-over, so you'll be more fun to be around! Not only that, you'll be physically capable of enjoying the beautiful scenic outdoors, you'll look better, younger and slimmer and be fitter. You'll feel better about yourself and that can translate into better and more frequent sex!

And of course, Sonja can also benefit from the Plan, because if she follows the eating program, her body will appreciate and respond to the low fat diet as well. She may already be naturally slim, but fat can still build up in slim people's arteries, and slim people can still feel bloated and sluggish after eating junk food. So trust me when I say, if you are fit and happy, your partner benefits in many ways as well.

As for the disabled transportation and adult diapers, Mike, you crack me up. Yes, I do agree that this example is the epitome of laziness. I admire the bloke's deviant creativity, but I detest his laziness. We all know that Americans do tend to make the headlines for doing some very odd things (no offence, Mike!). If Mother Nature gave us legs, feet, a heart and lungs that all work as they should, then people, let's use them for what they were intended!

Day 20. Half-Way to Health

> *Believe you can and you're halfway there.*
>
> – Theodore Roosevelt

Day 20…amazingly, I am halfway there.

It is coming on 1am, and for some reason I just cannot sleep. So it's me and my computer burning the midnight oil, while Sonja is in the land of nod. Hopefully I will join her there soon.

Early today, Sonja and I made the trek down to Bondi Beach for the Bondi-Coogee run, which I believe is 6.5 kilometres. And what an amazing view. Sonja and I soon split at about the 500 metre mark because she was keen to walk. At the gym, I usually need my iPod in order to avoid treadmill boredom, but outdoors with the waves, the sun, the noise of the sea…it's a sensory delight that makes exercising so much easier.

It was during this run that I realised I'd made some noticeable improvements in my fitness. There is a spot just south of Bronte Beach with a road that is straight uphill which leads to a seaside cemetery. Not long ago, that hill seriously punished me. If I wasn't bent over with my hands on my knees, I was slowly walking up with my heart beating a million times a minute. At the top of the hill, I would use the view of the ocean as an excuse to catch my breath for five minutes. But today was unprecedented. I wouldn't say I *attacked* the hill, but for the first time, the hill did not beat me. Certainly my pace slowed, but I kept my head up, shortened my steps, and I made it to the top at a pretty decent stride. And then, without stopping to check out the view at the top, I continued on my way.

I really am starting to become fit.

I'd left my gear at the gym, so I rewarded my performance with a nice steam, shave and shower. I felt fresh but was absolutely starving and needed some energy in a hurry.

Some mates were meeting down at the pub, which created a first-time dilemma in my City Caveman Plan – *caveman food versus pub food*. I had my brown bread chicken sandwich waiting for me at home, but to ditch the pub lunch and be anti-social would have been a bit rude on my part. So, Sonja and I headed down to Paddington for a pub lunch. A pint of lager would have gone down so nicely, but it was a big pint of water with a fresh squeeze of lime that I ordered instead. And then, the food battle hit me head on.

The pub menu came out.

Fried calamari, wedges with sour cream, regular fries, fish and chips, sirloin with Café de Paris butter on top, creamy pasta, and the list continued.

The choices were endless, and I so badly wanted the deep fried fish and chips. But I said no. There weren't a lot of options for the health-conscious, but I managed to find an option of grilled chicken with pumpkin. And, I must say, it was fantastic.

Normally I would have had numerous beers, fish and all-of-the-chips, had that bloated food-coma feeling, and gone home for a Saturday afternoon snooze. But after my choices today I felt fantastic. A few waters, good conversation, a couple of laughs and a very tasty chicken dish saw me leaving the bar in the same state I arrived: fresh, healthy and feeling good.

Definitely a lesson learned; not every meal out has to be a pig-out session full of greasy, fried flavours. I still came home and had a great nanna nap, but at least this time it was because of a run, rather than being in a fatty-food coma.

Caveman Tip:

No matter the situation, stick with the City Caveman Eating Plan. From the fast-food spots to the fish and chip shops, *there are healthy options*, you just have to look a little harder to find them.

Sonja and I had a birthday party to go to in the evening, so we ventured out for another night of social non-drinking, which was difficult, but my friend's compliment of 'Wow, your skin is glowing,' made me feel kind of good about myself and what I was doing. I mean, as a guy, when a girl says 'Wow, your skin looks great,' I'm not entirely sure how to respond, but I thanked her and, hey, if my skin does look better, then I guess I must look a bit younger and that can only be a good thing. I am never that good at accepting compliments, especially when they're so…personal? Her Scottish boyfriend was heading to the bar, so he asked what I was drinking – 'Just a water, mate,' I said. And with that came the onslaught of another battle.

Rejecting a drink from a Scotsman is a serious no-no. The chap was already half cut, so he took on the responsibility of busting my chops every three minutes by declaring, 'The Yank will have another pussy-water.' Oh well. I knew being a City Caveman wasn't going to be easy.

There was a moment that night, where I was chatting with Sonja and was entirely drink-less. It felt strangely uncomfortable because I was not holding anything and so I kind of didn't know what to do with my hands. I think smokers who have recently quit have this issue as well; they don't know what to do with their free hand when it's not grasping a cigarette. It was a funny sensation; it actually makes me look forward to my first wine after Day 40.

Over the past 20 days, it has been so nice to be able to enjoy the sun, the outdoors, the fresh air, nice runs, the ocean, the non-hangover mornings, a clear mind and fresh, tasty, healthy food. And it's not just been *nice*, but it has been a *nice change*. Instead of planning drinks, drinks, drinks all weekend, I am planning days in the sun, at the beach, and tomorrow is no different. Tomorrow we are going for a nice Sunday walk in Manly. I have made a shift from being a night creature to one who enjoys making morning plans that involve a run, a walk and a healthy meal. Life is becoming much, much nicer in the Caveman's world.

So, as I sign off on the halfway mark, do I have any new reflections? No, not really. I wish I had some grand advice or philosophical saying to commemorate the first half of my journey or to inspire me for the second half, but I don't.

The only thing I should do is clarify that 'I' am not halfway there, but 'we' are halfway there. I could not be doing this without Annie's advice, guidance and support. She has successfully put up with my moans and groans and has continued to motivate me every time I need a little pep talk.

It's been twenty days of battles, and twenty days of wins. I'm ready to take on twenty more, and I'm ready to battle on until I find that place where health and change is finally mine.

Annie's say: *Halfway there! I am so happy! We have made it this far, and we only have to continue and build on what we have done for the last twenty days in order to succeed! Hang in there, Mikey. It's all cruising downhill from here on – psychologically speaking, that is. Physically, I will still be whipping your arse into shape as hard as I ever have!*

I am glad to hear that Mike is feeling fitter and those hill runs are seeming easier. For everybody making a healthy change, the fitter you become, the greater your feelings of self-esteem and confidence. Fitness and confidence do go hand-in-hand,

and I think it's pretty obvious that, when you are feeling good and looking good, confidence levels go through the roof! And of course, a boost in self-esteem and confidence can filter through to other areas of your life, making it better in lots of ways. The mental and physical changes you will receive at the end of the City Caveman Plan are endless!

And a final 'well done' to Mike on managing to find a healthy option from a bar menu. Alcohol is usually served with fatty, fried foods at a bar, so I'm glad to hear that Mike managed to avoid this potential stumbling block and have a healthy chicken meal with his water. However, it sounds to me like Mike is feeling like a bit of a nerd drinking water among the drinking folk – especially around a Scotsman – so why not branch out and have a juice? I recommend cranberry or tomato. They are a bit more exciting than water but still healthy, and can be less conspicuous, so you might be able to avoid a few of the friendly insults.

With all the exercise in the sun, skin glowing and no hangovers, Mike sounds in a very positive frame of mind. It is good to know the Caveman lifestyle is bringing out the best in him. I hope we achieve as much in the next twenty days as we have from the first twenty, and when that euphoria wears off, we will hang in there together and just stick to the Plan. We've made it this far, Mike, so we can definitely make it the whole way. Just keep staying focused, battle, win and enjoy the healthy challenges each day brings!

13

City Caveman Days 21 to 30 – *Finding the Groove*

Day 21. Dieting

> *I've been on a diet for two weeks and all I've lost is fourteen days.*
>
> – Totie Fields

Sunday: my happy day off. I had a grand sleep-in today and woke up fresh as a daisy. Sonja and I headed off to Manly for a nice little beach/bush walk on a perfect 23-degree day.

I was thinking again about the party last night. I remember chatting with a girl about my City Caveman Plan. She was curious and interested to know what I ate, how I felt, etc., but she kept saying 'diet' and talking about 'dieting', which really got annoying after a while because the City Caveman Plan is NOT a diet.

I know I expressed my feelings about dieting earlier, but with there being so many schemes, fads and lies out there, it's worth echoing the point that diets are simply useless, and I think the following information that I found online[iv] is worth reading:

iv Wolpert, Stuart, 2007, 'Dieting Does Not Work, UCLA Researchers Report', <http://www.newsroom.ucla.edu/portal/ucla/Dieting-Does-Not-Work-UCLA-Researchers-7832.aspx?RelNum=7832>.

Dieting Does Not Work, Researchers Report

'You can initially lose 5 to 10 per cent of your weight on any number of diets, but then the weight comes back,' said Traci Mann, UCLA associate professor of psychology and lead author of the study. 'We found that the majority of people regained all the weight, plus more. Sustained weight loss was found only in a small minority of participants, while complete weight regain was found in the majority. Diets do not lead to sustained weight loss or health benefits for the majority of people.'

Mann and her co-authors conducted the most comprehensive and rigorous analysis of diet studies, analysing 31 long-term studies.

'What happens to people on diets in the long run?' Mann asked. 'Would they have been better off to not go on a diet at all? We decided to dig up and analyse every study that followed people on diets for two to five years. We concluded most of them would have been better off not going on the diet at all. Their weight would be pretty much the same, and their bodies would not suffer the wear and tear from losing weight and gaining it all back.'

And further down in that article…

If dieting doesn't work, what does?

'Eating in moderation is a good idea for everybody, and so is regular exercise,' Mann said. 'That is not what we looked at in this study. Exercise may well be the key factor leading to sustained weight loss. Studies consistently find that people who reported the most exercise also had the most weight loss.'

Evidence suggests that repeatedly losing and gaining weight is linked to cardiovascular disease, stroke, diabetes and altered immune function. Mann and Tomiyama recommend that more research be conducted on the health effects of losing and gaining weight, noting that scientists do not fully understand how such weight cycling leads to adverse health effects.

Caveman Tip:

Never, ever go on a *diet*, as

a diets suck, and they are boring;

b diets do not work; and,

c yo-yo dieting leads to serious health problems in the long-term.

I am continuing to ignore the diet trends and put my faith in the City Caveman Plan because it revolves around healthy, balanced and tasty meals to provide energy, while still allowing for fat loss. Perfect!

Another article I found during my research process[v] addressed obesity levels in Australia. A snippet of this is below:

Report on the Childhood Obesity Summit

The incidence of childhood and adolescent obesity has trebled over the last decade. Many of these children progress into adult obesity. Currently over half of our adult population is overweight or obese. New disorders presenting in obese adolescents include type 2 diabetes, hypertension, hyperlipidaemia, fatty liver, sleep apnoea, asthma, orthopaedic complications including postural imbalance and excessive weight bearing, and poorer psychosocial functioning and reduced self-esteem levels.

Child obesity in Australia? With so many parks, beaches and outdoor areas and such a strong sporting culture, how can this happen? Families and politicians have tried to lay blame on external influences, such as fast food advertising during children's television hours, but that's bullshit. I've never known a seven-year-old who sees an advertisement on television to grab the car keys and drive to the store for an unhealthy food purchase. If kids are eating junk food, then it's the parent's fault isn't it? Be a good parent, do the right thing and feed your children healthy meals.

If we really want to arrest obesity in kids, I say just turn the television off altogether, give them a soccer ball, sign them up for community sports and

---

v Trigger, Dr. Robert, 2002, 'Report on the Childhood Obesity Summit, <http://www.medicineau.net.au/clinical/obesity/obesit2271.html>.

switch off their computers and Nintendos. Sports are played outdoors with mates while running and moving about, not indoors with remote controls and televisions.

With regard to children suffering from adult conditions, such as diabetes, heart conditions or back problems, it has to be an example of the *roll-down effect*, which is a made-up term I use when referring to the fact that children are extremely affected and influenced by their parents. I mean, seriously, would a triathlete husband and wife have an obese child? They eat healthy and fresh food, snack sensibly and are accountable for what goes into their body, so that is what they will teach their child. There is a natural roll-down effect. Of course, as the child gets older and they can make their own decisions, things can change, but in those formative years, attentive parents will tend to lay the foundations for a child's outlook toward food and health.

We all have choices, we all have options and, while we are all influenced by marketing to a degree, what we put into our bodies is ultimately up to us.

***Annie says**: I love both these articles.*

In the first article, I particularly like the quote 'Exercise may well be the key factor leading to sustained fat loss.' How many times do we need to say this? It's so true! And so simple! Just like we've already said: do not EVER starve yourself or go on stupid fad diets. Get active, people! Our bodies are designed to be exercised on a regular basis, so walk instead of taking the car, bus or train; take the stairs instead of the elevator; ride a bike; even a stationary bike in front of the television is an okay option if that's all you can manage. Don't be a spectator – be a participant. It's way more fun and your body will thank you for it.

I also agree with Mike's point about childhood obesity and the fact that parents need to take responsibility for their child's health. It's true that kids are exposed to advertising, but it is the parents who have the money, so it is the parents who are responsible for what food is purchased and, ultimately, consumed. How about you just don't buy fast food, lollies, chips, soft drinks, ice-cream and chocolate? Or, let them have those things once in a while as a treat, but do not give it to them all the time. Obesity, and its many associated diseases, are all preventable and the old adage is true: prevention is better than cure, so let's start taking steps to prevent the continuation of this obesity epidemic, rather than jumping on the yo-yo diet bandwagon in a bid to cure it.

Day 22. My Tattoo

> *We all have the ability...we just don't all have the courage to follow our dreams and to follow the signs.*
>
> – Paulo Coelho

It was kind of an up and down day for me today.

Up because I had a good day at the gym, and I was really cruising. Mentally I am really starting to push it. The only downside is that I risk complacency, which has the potential to lead to laziness, which isn't good! So, I am going to try stepping up my workouts a bit. The weights are still a challenge, so I am going to pick up my running as well, not too much, but today I ran an extra two minutes prior to my upper body workout, and starting tomorrow I will also try to increase the run during my cardio-only days.

And it was *down* because...well, I don't actually know. Maybe I'm over-thinking it, but today I was wondering if I really will be able to continue a healthy life beyond the 40-day target.

As I write this, one of my very favourite books is sitting right under my feet. *The Alchemist* is written by Paulo Coehlo. It's a beautiful tale about Santiago, a Spanish shepherd who has a dream and also has the courage to follow it. After listening to *the signs* the boy travels into Africa for a journey of self-discovery, adventure, risks and reward. What I love most about this book is the way the author uses signs and symbols throughout the story and how Santiago always takes the time to notice these signs and let them guide him during his journey.

On a personal level, this notion really strikes a chord because in my pre-City Caveman Plan days, not only had I stopped thinking and listening to my body, but I had also stopped seeing its signs. They were all there, plain for me and everyone else to see; my waistline, my belly, my chubby face, those photos...and the most important sign of all: my tattoo.

People get tattoos for many reasons, some due to drunkenness, but usually for a more significant or deeper purpose. Tattoos are signs, symbols and reminders. And what really bothers me about myself was that I missed the most obvious sign, even though I saw it every single day when I looked in the mirror.

I was an active, healthy kid with no real medical problems until I was about seven years old. It started with a little bit of pain in my right shoulder, which then turned into a noticeable lump a few days later. My poor mum and dad were, as you'd expect, terrified. I was equally as scared, of course, especially having to see the distinct look of worry in my parents' eyes.

Thankfully, the lump revealed itself to be a scare only, but after a week in the hospital and stressful surgery, I was left with a permanent war-wound, in an eight-by-two centimetre long scar on my right shoulder: my *tattoo*.

So for my entire adult life I have had this visually prominent reminder on my arm of how precious my health can be. It's there for me to see every day, but I have essentially stopped taking notice what this sign truly means.

I suppose that's where some of today's concern stems from; will I remember to look out for the signs after my forty days are over?

Caveman Tip:

Signs are everywhere in our lives. If we take note of them, they can be useful as guides to remember the journey in life we should be taking.

So, I need to make a conscious effort from here on, to recognise those signs more often. To look at my own special mark of luck and remember how fortunate I am to actually have been given that second chance to live a healthy life.

Annie says: *Short and sweet from me today, because I think Mike said it all.*

Signs and symbols can be amazing reminders as well as motivators in one's life. But it's always a case of 'do you stop and take notice of these signs, or do you disregard and overlook them and not invest the time to understand what they actually mean in your life?'

For Mike, his sign of health was right there throughout the years, yet he refused to take notice. A bit late but not too late, Mike has finally realised the deeper meaning of his tattoo. And from now on, this self-realisation of what that mark truly means will always look different to him; it is his permanent sign to guide him in his healthy, post-City Caveman Plan days.

Day 23. Smoking Sucks

> *Cancer cures smoking.*
>
> – Author unknown

It's the middle of Sydney winter, but today was 24 degrees! Needless to say, I felt quite cheery on my way into the gym today.

The entrance to my gym has about forty stairs to climb, which, not *that* long ago, used to reliably steal my breath from me. Yet today, I bounced my way up those stairs, and just as I was nearing the top, I passed a chap on his way out who had an unlit cigarette hanging out of his mouth.

Now, I've seen folks act like drunken morons at bars, sports fans behaving like morons at the cricket pitch, and we have all heard of the double burger with cheese and bacon followed up with a 'Diet Coke please', but to see an idiot walk out of the gym after just having worked out getting ready to light up a cancer stick – it's disgusting.

I know the look he was trying to convey; that 'I'm so cool and rebellious that I can even smoke after coming out of the gym' look. Is he a rebel? A tool, more like it!

Well, it is his body and, therefore, his choice. Maybe I should just chill out a bit and let him enjoy his slow death. Or, maybe I should have shared these facts with him:[vi]

- **a** A former Russian spy was allegedly murdered using Plutonium-210. This radioactive chemical is also found in cigarette smoke, a fact at least one tobacco company was aware of in 1964.
- **b** In 1989, millions of cases of imported fruit were banned after a small amount of cyanide was found in just two grapes. There's 33 times more cyanide in a single cigarette than was found in both of those grapes.
- **c** Hydrogen cyanide has been used in prison executions. It's also found in cigarette smoke.
- **d** Sodium hydroxide is a caustic compound found in hair removal products. It's also found in cigarettes.
- **e** Soups, cereals and other products we consume have to list ingredients on their labels, but cigarettes – which are estimated to contribute to killing a third of their users – are not required to list any of the 599 additives.

Whether you smoke at home, at the bar or walking out of the gym, the bottom line is: you're not a rebel, you're a fool.

Smoking annoys me. I simply don't understand it. But, maybe, it comes from my family background. Mum has never touched a cigarette in her life, while Dad nearly invented chain smoking at three to four packs a day, so my home environment had the two extremes.

I am proud to say that I have never been tempted to see what the *less oxygen, more poisonous smoke* lifestyle was like. In fact, I have never even put a cigarette in my mouth – ever. Sonja thinks I fart enough as it is and that, as a result, I inhale enough noxious gas without needing to fork over $12 a pack for it.

After passing Smokey at the gym, I assumed my Game Day approach and prepared to take my battle stance against my cardio workout, with extra minutes added on because I want to start pushing my body a little harder.

---

vi TheTruth.com Facts, 2007, <www.TheTruth.com>.

It wasn't too long ago that I would want to do something physically, yet my body was incapable of doing it. I could increase my time in the shower, bar or on the couch by many minutes, but on the treadmill? No way. However, today, it was a breeze! I just zoned out and before I knew it, my time was up. And so, another battle was won.

Caveman Tip:

If you're feeling healthy and fit and your body can handle it, increase the time and/or intensity of your City Caveman workouts.

I am starting to feel that my mind and body are up for mental and physical challenges that would previously have been too much for me.

The City Caveman Plan has no hangovers, no bloated tummy and no food coma, just a hankering to up the ante and really start to challenge myself, both mentally and physically.

Now, although my body is responding well at the gym in terms of my fitness levels and how I feel, I am still a bit concerned about my actual body *shape*. Thankfully, a supportive email from Annie helped relieve my 'shape anxiety'. She wrote:

> *Don't get caught up so much with your perceived shape. You have stuck to the eating plan, and with all the exercise you are doing your body is shifting body fat to muscle weight, so relax. Will check you out tomorrow but you were looking slimmer last time I saw you, so I'm sure you're still on track.*

Shit. I hope I check out okay tomorrow. Good looking gym girls don't usually give my body the up-and-down (well, not favourably), and now Annie is going to suss me out. I hope she keeps the pointing and giggles to a minimum.

So, you might recall I mentioned how critical my iPod is to my cardio training in the gym? Well, here's my tip of the day:

> *iPods are not meant to fluff, tumble, nor go through the spin cycle.*

Damn it! I bought an iPod Shuffle a few months back and today I forgot to take it off the back of my running shirt, and so there it went, through the wash cycle and into the tumble dryer. And then into the rubbish bin!

But, like life, it's all about attitude and the silver lining of this loss was that I get to buy myself a new one!

So, iPod aside, all in all I had a good day in the cave today. Sonja interviewed for her first Aussie job and got it on the spot. So, dinner is on me tonight, and I will treat her to a post-dinner champagne. The Austrian Devil can indulge in her choice of Asian delights and white wine, while I will stick to my water with a plate of brown rice, steamed veggies and chicken with my signature splash of soy!

So, congratulations to Sonja on her new job. I am looking forward to winning tomorrow's battles, which include a tough workout with Annie, and although today wasn't all thumbs up, it is still sunny in the Caveman world.

Annie says*: I am totally with you on the anti-smoking. I tried it once, hated it and have never smoked again. Neither of my parents smoked and neither do the majority of my friends. It's an unhealthy, disgusting habit that causes lung cancer and too many other illnesses to name here. With all the evidence that cigarettes kill and the gross pictures on the packet, I don't know how anyone can resist fighting the addiction.*

If you're a smoker, please make the change. In fact, make giving up smoking your first goal to a better life. By being a non-smoker, you will get so much more out of both the City Caveman Plan and life itself.

Day 24. Conquering My Mount Everest

It is not the mountains that we conquer, but ourselves.

– Sir Edmund Hillary

While I was working in New York some years back, I remember watching an evening news special, which featured a story on Mount Everest where two separate groups of climbers tried to reach the summit. Unfortunately, the weather, altitude, time and supplies of oxygen all worked against them and eight people perished during the expedition. One of the survivors, Jon Krakauer, later wrote *Into Thin Air* detailing his experience, and I highly recommend it for anyone seeking inspiration and an amazing adventure story.

The book is one of my favourites, but I remember the news story really well because, while it aired, my father called me from Chicago, and this would turn out to be the last conversation I would ever have with him.

Around that time I was actually travelling back and forth between Chicago and New York as part of a consulting job I was doing. At the same time Dad was in and out of the hospital due to fluctuating health. After my week of transient work, I headed back toward Chicago and, during my stay, I got the call. Dad was only alive because of the machines he had been hooked up to, and this was a situation that our family had agreed we would not prolong if it ever arose.

Of course, this was the most emotionally difficult and overwhelming day of my life. To see, hear and watch my dad pass on was devastating. It was, at least, some comfort to have our whole family there to say goodbye and support each other through the grief.

So for me, the last dialogue I had with my dad was during the airing of that Everest special. Every day since his passing my dad pops into my thoughts; sometimes it's a conscious thought of missing him, sometimes something evokes a memory of him, and sometimes it's me consciously wishing I could have just one more marathon dinner with him in Chicago.

And today was no different; today Dad popped into my thoughts.

I went over to Annie's house for today's workout, because Hunter was still a little unwell. We did yet another good leg workout, and even managed to mix it up a little with some 'holding the baby' moves! To keep Hunter happy, we decided that when one of us would do the leg workout, the other would hold Hunter, and then we'd switch and pass the baby. Now, in my time, I've passed the wine and passed the crème sauce, but until now, I'd never passed the baby – it was a neat experience!

When Hunter finally fell asleep, Annie and I strapped him in and went running in the park. It was a perfect day for it, so instead of doing our usual two laps around the park, after the first one Annie said, 'Hey, let's do some running over at the hill.' *Note to every reader: When your trainer says the word 'hill', stop talking and stop smiling, because you are in for it.*

So, after a slow lazy jog, we came upon 'the hill'. The first thing that came to my mind when I looked up at that hill was, 'holy shit'. Annie said, 'What I want is simple: sprint up that hill five times. You can catch your breath on the jog down.' My mind repeated itself. 'Holy shit.' The battle was not only the hill, which I promptly christened *Mount Holy Shit*, but there were actually hills within the hill – namely, three of them. The drawing below details what I was looking at:

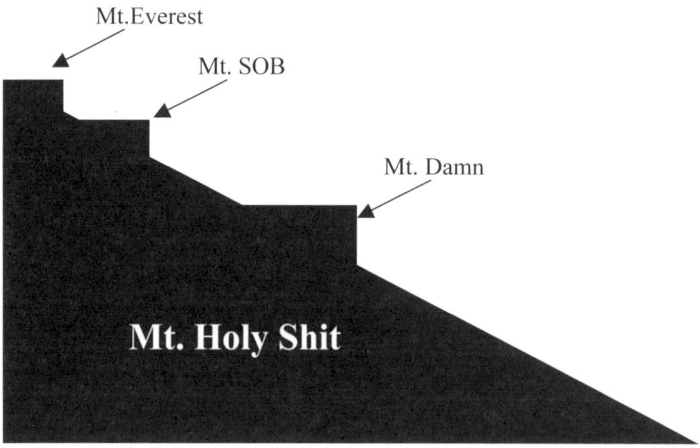

By the time I reached the top, I was panting like a beer-drinking marathon runner, hands on my knees, legs like jelly. I was right in the middle of figuring out ways to subtly delay the downward leg so I could squeeze in more recovery time, when I hear Annie (who I now don't like very much) yell, 'One down, four to go.'

'Holy shit.'

As you can imagine, the next three trips up and down that hill were bloody challenging and, to the casual observer, Annie, Hunter and I probably looked like a husband-wife-son combination, with the wife holding the son yelling at the cursing husband to run faster up and down Mount Holy Shit. What a wacky scene. On my fourth trip down the hill, I found myself thinking how much I wanted a beer. Yet, right as my thoughts were wandering to the golden ale, Annie chirped in with, 'Mike, use your mind as well as your body. On your last trip up at that hill, I want you to say over and over in your mind, 'I am fit, I am fit, I am fit.'

'Holy shit.'

My fifth battle up that hill was definitely my best effort. But I must admit, the 'I am fit' thing only got me half the way up. During certain hardships, I think all of us have a tendency to draw upon songs, feelings, thoughts or people to motivate us, whether they be emotionally tough times or physical challenges. For me, after I crossed Mount Damn, I conjured up the memory of my father for inspiration. Oddly, I thought of my father at the top of this Mount Everest, holding the end of a rope with the other end tied around my waist. And he was pulling me. And, as a result, my arms pumped harder, my knees moved faster and I got up my personal Mount Everest in my best time yet.

After that fifth summit scaling, I was so tired I had to zigzag down rather than walk in a straight line and make my thighs cry. Annie was talking to me at the time, but I didn't actually hear her. I was still thinking about Dad and our awesome joint effort. And to add a little more wow to the Dad-Everest connection, when I got home, the Discovery Channel was airing the final episode of the *Everest* documentary. Today's occurrences brought me a bit closer than normal to my dad. It was a pretty great feeling.

Caveman Tip:

Deep down, each of us has a motivating influence. Find yours. It will help you run that extra kilometre, lift that last rep and climb that final stair.

***Annie says**: I'm not quite sure about naming the hill 'Holy Shit' because we don't want to offend anyone. But, in thinking back to that hill, I have to agree that only a swear word will do!*

I cried, I laughed and I was inspired by Mike's writing today. I'm sorry to hear of the loss of his father as, having lost my mother to cancer, I know first-hand that nothing compares to the loss of a parent you love. I also think of my mother every day, especially now that I have Hunter. And, like Mike, thoughts of her have inspired me to conquer my own personal Mount Everests.

Constant conquering of physical challenges not only improves your physicality, but it also strengthens your character, which means that you are able to deal with emotional challenges a little easier too.

I can understand how the visualisation of Mike's dad pulling him to the top of that hill would inspire him to achieve the challenge put before him. I am also sure that Mike's dad would have been feeling very proud of his son for giving it his all in this quest to become a better, healthier man.

I encourage you to follow Mike's example and use thoughts of your loved ones to help you make it through the tough challenges. Getting fit and becoming healthy isn't, after all, just about you, remember? In the bigger picture, your health affects everyone in your world; your work, your social life, your loved ones. And, of course, the healthier you are, the longer you will live, and those who need you will benefit not only from your increased energy and wellbeing but also your longevity.

Now, I must thank Mike again for his patience with my son. He was being very diplomatic when he forgot to mention that he was screaming like a banshee for much of our workout, and anyone less patient would have taken the first bus out of there! I must say, though, it was very cute to see him playing dad between each set of leg exercises. Although I'm not too sure about the cursing part!

Anyone, from mothers to business executives, who claim they don't have time to work out can no longer use that excuse. You do have time, you just have to be a little flexible and creative about how and where you train. Of course, this highlights the importance of finding an understanding training partner as well.

Even though we had a workout that was, literally, all over the place today, I really enjoyed training with Mike. See? We trainers also reap the rewards from working with our clients. We had a great leg workout in my tiny gym, a leisurely run around the park, and I was so pleased with Mike's effort in running up that hill not once, but FIVE times. 'Fat Mike' is so gone! He really is 'Fit Mike' now!

Today leaves me looking forward to our leg workout next week. So how about we aim for ten times up that hill?

Day 25. Corporate Marketing Machines

> *Companies spend billions to make sure that you know their product. In 2001, on direct media advertising – that's radio, television and print – McDonald's spent $1.4 billion worldwide. On direct media advertising, Pepsi spent more than a billion dollars. To advertise candy, Hershey foods spent a mere $200 million internationally. In its peak year the 'Five-a-Day Vegetable Campaigns' total advertising budget in all media was a lowly $2 million, a hundred times less than just the direct media budget of one candy company.*
>
> – Morgan Spurlock, Super Size Me

Ohhhhhhh, this morning I really felt the effects of Mount Everest in my hamstrings, my bum and even my feet! Changing our workout like that was a damn good idea and my body knows it! Another Caveman lesson learned: *the body will become used to what you throw at it. And when it does, you amp it up!*

Annie did check out my body yesterday before our run and I am happy to say she confirmed that I have slimmed down quite a lot. Also, she said my skin is making me look a lot younger than before! Woohoo! But, seriously, it is strange how I misperceive myself. Still. In my eyes I still see a chubby man, yet others are commenting on my weight loss.

Maybe it is a case of familiarity? I see my eyes in the mirror, and since they don't change, the whole package surrounding those eyes must not be changing either. Okay, I don't know.

I have refrained from stepping on the scales, heeding that initial advice from Annie, so I don't know what my true fat loss is at this point. But, I guess I will just keep plugging along and trust that the process we have planned will get me to my desired destination. Hell, I really do feel great. And it helps to hear that I look better too. What a great motivator!

You know what though? I am beginning to think that the body is not that complex after all. I mean, it's kind of like a simple recipe, where if you mix ingredients X with Y and Z, you will create a nice meal. The body is similar; if you restrict your intake of fat to X grams and couple it with healthy Y nutrients, and then you add an effective exercise plan, the body *will* respond the way you want it to. It's simple.

I was in Blockbuster recently, when I saw a woman in her mid-20s. With no offence to her, she really looked exhausted. Picture it. She held a one-year-old baby with her right arm, a handful of DVDs in her right hand, her six-year-old daughter was at her side clutching onto her left hand, and her five-year-old son was bouncing around the shop like he had just spent the week in a sugar factory – and it was only 6pm! And just like crowds chant their favourite football team's name in the last remaining seconds of a match, the boy started pulling at his Mom's trousers, yelling, 'MILKY BAR, MILKY BAR, MILKY BAR!' He was holding one of those huge blocks that I'm sure were designed to feed a small army. His mum replied, 'No, no; please put those back.' He replied, 'Mummy, mummy, I want Milky Bar,' to which she replied, 'No son, those are not good for you.' His response? 'But no mummy look – they have *milk* in them!' I couldn't help myself from laughing. How could a mum say no to a witty response like that?

The point of this story is that people respond to marketing. As much as we may not like it, the truth is that we are affected by advertising messages. I truly feel for families who suffer at the hands of the marketing conglomerates who plaster those horrible, sugary cereals with the latest animated character or celebrity in a bid to attract the children. The sad thing is: it works! Furthermore, they use deceptive product names, like *Froot* Loops, which makes them sound healthy despite the fact that three cups pack a massive 39 grams of sugar (the US daily recommendation is only 40 grams!).

Caveman Tip:

Corporations spend fortunes tempting our eyes and taste buds. Be smart, look at labels and take responsibility for what you put into your stomach as well as your children's.

So, from 'milk' chocolate to 'froot' cereals, I just need to be mindful and alert to what is catching my consumer eye. Sure, a little chocolate would be a nice treat right now, but the City Caveman Plan is just the therapy I need to get my health and my life back on track.

Annie says: *We are more than three weeks into the Plan now and Mike is definitely reaping the rewards from his great eating and solid workouts. The change is definitely noticeable. In fact, he is starting to look amazing! Whether he is conscious of it or not, he is much leaner, his eyes sparkle and his skin glows. I am so excited for all of us to view the 'after' photos once that fortieth day arrives! Maybe then he will be able to compare them to the 'before' photos and see for himself how much he has really improved.*

As I said earlier, it is hard to see subtle differences when you eye yourself off every day, but I am certain that comparing the 'before' and 'after' photos will have a big impact on Mike and the way he sees himself. I think after the comparison he will be able to see the change that others are already seeing in him.

As for Milky Bars and Froot Loops, I just have three things to say: crap, crap and more crap. Skip the marketing schemes and see things for what they really are. The beauty of the City Caveman Plan is the detailed Plan that actually tells you exactly what you need and what you need to do to become fit, lean and healthy. We've not added any wacky slogans or recruited any cash-for-comment style endorsements. The City Caveman Plan is all about fresh fruit and vegetables, lean protein and regular exercise. Simple, simple, simple and, as Mike is discovering, very, very effective.

Day 26. Stairway to...Hell

There is no elevator to success. You have to take the stairs.

– Author unknown

I think Annie is trying to kill me. Or she must really be getting me into good shape.

My directions for today were to swap my chest workout for a run, warm up on my own and meet her at the dog park down at Coogee Beach. Thankfully it was another gorgeous Sydney day and after the warm-up run, I went to my favourite juice shop and bought a piece of pineapple before meeting Annie, Hunter and their dog, Bam Bam. When Annie saw me, she looked at my bigger-than-a-brick sized portion of pineapple and said, 'What's that?'

'Pineapple. Want some?

'No, and you're crazy cause that is not going to sit well in your stomach.'

'Bah, I'll be fine. I thought a little fruit-sugar kick would be good for me.'

'Okaaaaaaaaay. Let's go then,' she said.

'Where to?'

'You'll see.'

We jogged down a beautiful path to a location that was new to me, and we stopped right in front of the most hellishly steep stairs I'd ever seen. These stairs made Mount Holy Shit look like an ant hill.

Mental note: Annie's surprises are not necessarily good.

So, up and down we went, five times each way. And with stairs, there is absolutely no possibility of cheating or faking it. The running belt on a treadmill *moves to* the runner, so you can semi-cheat when you're running on one. Similarly, the stairs on a stairmaster move with the climber, so you can semi-cheat on a gym-based stair run too. But with real stairs? Forget it.

Clearly, Bam Bam was the only one excited to be there.

From the bottom, you are able to see where they flatten out. Only, it turns out that when you get to that flat part, it's actually flat for about 30 metres before you are faced with another wall of stairs. At that flat part, you're only halfway there. Shit. This was not exercise. It was torture.

I know that right now I am whingeing like a child but, believe me, had I any breath to whinge while on the stairs, I would have. Every muscle in my legs was being worked simultaneously, and the cardio workout was equally extraordinary. My heart was pumping like crazy, and my legs were taking a beating as I carried my body weight up and down all 218 stairs.

Annie's directions were to keep moving. Damn her. The only respite I received from the leg pain was during the brief moments when I reached the top, where I got a well-earned reward in the amazing, expansive ocean views.

And then it hit me – that damn pineapple. It was now gurgling in my stomach and causing me some digestion-related issues. I was mid-pant, struggling through my third summit, when I felt it coming. My mouth was dry, but it soon had saliva in it, and I knew right then and there that the pineapple was coming.

Without a choice, I hurled over the stair railing. I'll refrain from sharing too much detail, but at least it didn't go on beyond one episode. I stopped for a few seconds, looked for Annie or anybody for a bit of sympathy, but I got nothing. All I could do was keep on moving.

If those stairs were an Olympic event, I was definitely contending for the bronze medal. While I was huffing and puffing, Annie was carrying eight kilogram Hunter on her shoulder sling, which was an amazing feat. She couldn't be happy whizzing her own lithe body up those stairs, she had to go and add on another bundle for extra resistance! Impressively, Hunter actually fell asleep in his little shoulder pouch, so Annie softened each of her steps to ensure he wouldn't be woken up by the motion.

I made five rounds of those stairs, and Annie made four while holding a sleeping baby – quite an effort, if I do say so myself!

And as for Bam Bam? I swear I would not be shocked if he ran on batteries. The height of every one of those steps was 75 per cent the size of his own body, yet he was ALL OVER the stairs, sometimes following me, sometimes following Annie. Bam Bam was acting like he didn't know which way was up or down and, in the end, he must have done the equivalent of seven full rounds of those stairs.

At the end Annie said, 'Mike, you conquered the stairs', to which I replied, 'I'm not sure "conquer" is the word I would use, unless you want to say that the stairs conquered me!'

Between Mount Holy Shit and the newly named Stairway to Hell, I realise that the improvements on my fitness levels will have escalated so much faster with this type of training, than if I'd just kept running on that (semi-cheat) treadmill.

Caveman Tip:

The City Caveman Workout is *not* set in stone. Listen to your body and seek out new challenges. New methods of training are a great way to physically feed your body something different.

***Annie says**: I knew that pineapple would come back up again! Here he is, Caveman Mike, about to embark on a training session, and he's eating pineapple. Is he crazy? Do you see any Olympic runners munching on pineapple before a big race? No! Maybe next time he will take me more seriously and come prepared – with an empty stomach!*

Well done, Mike, on conquering the Coogee stairs five times – even though you did have a chuck in the middle. And yes, you DID conquer them!

To me, those stairs are a good measure of fitness, and anyone who can do them five times is pretty fit in my books, so Mike has definitely come a long way.

In Week 1, I don't think Mike could have walked up the stairs once, let alone run up them five times in a row.

And thanks to him for acknowledging my four times. The things we mothers have to do to get our babies to sleep! He did look like a little angel though. And my little Wonder Pooch, Bam Bam! He's so bouncy and light on his feet and I tell you: those stairs are one of the few things that really tire him out.

So, I've thrown Mike two curveballs in the past week, with the hill and stair training. And guess what? His mind and body coped very well. He is changing and he is learning to change fast now.

I cannot stress enough the importance of mixing up your training because, as Mike said, the body is smart and it adapts quickly to challenges. That means if you put it through the same workout all the time, your body will eventually stop reacting because it gets used to the load you are putting it under.

So, the secret to improving is change. Vary your workouts and you'll keep challenging yourself to greater Caveman victories.

Day 27. I Cheated

No one can cheat you out of ultimate success but yourself.

–Ralph Waldo Emerson

Yow, today I woke up a bit sore, but not really muscle soreness; it was more like general fatigue. The body was shot. I wonder why some days it comes but other days it doesn't? Friday's stairs definitely took their toll on my body, and today's workout was no easy feat. But, that's the Plan, right? Another day, another battle.

Yesterday was a running day, so today I had a back and chest workout and it was SLOW! What normally takes me an hour took me an extra 20 minutes. My warm-up run was slow, and so were my chest exercises. But, in the scheme of things it didn't matter, given that in the 'old' days a Saturday workout would have been negligible due to the effects of a hangover! So, if the battle is bigger today as a direct result of the Caveman Workout Plan, then that can only really be good news. And the fact I didn't ditch this workout altogether, well it's another victory won, really!

The good news of the day really had nothing to do with the gym but more to do with a shirt. Last Christmas when Sonja came for a visit, she gave me a super cool shirt as a present. It was one of those European-styled shirts with extended cuffs, wide and high collars and a print down the right side. It has a great tapered, V-shaped cut to it. It really was beautiful. But, unfortunately, at the time she gave it to me, the chub on my body didn't quite do that shirt justice. In fact, it didn't really fit well at all. The buttons and seams didn't fall nicely down the shirt; they were pulled to the sides as a result of chub-induced tension…it fit like a Speedo shirt. So, the shirt was quietly relegated to its hanger in the wardrobe, and that's where it had stayed ever since.

But today – what a victory! Today I put this shirt on, and it fit like a glove. (No, I didn't wear it on my hands!) It hung so perfectly and, in fact, I even had some room to spare. And if the fact I could wear it, and wear it well, wasn't enough reward, let's just say that Sonja really enjoyed seeing me in it. My new body is finally taking form (I think), and it's actually beginning to affect my style as well – great news.

It was such a great realisation to understand that this shirt fit me so well now because for the past 26 days, I have refrained from alcohol, my favourite cheeses, fizzy drinks, cheeky snacks, ice cream and unhealthy breakfasts. I have said 'no' at the outdoor drinking festivals, mates' birthday nights and nights out at the pub. Temptations and cravings have come and gone, with me winning the battles.

Except for tonight…

Tonight, for the first time, I fell off the City Caveman Plan. I cheated.

Sonja has been in Australia for a few weeks now, and we haven't yet shared a bottle of wine together or a meal without me making sure it had only Caveman ingredients. She has been a pretty good sport about it, but I can tell it has been a bit taxing on her. Monday is her 24th birthday, so tonight was our night to celebrate it together and, in my mind, the only way to celebrate a birthday is with good wine, great food and a giant splash of romance.

For our celebration, I found the perfect little Spanish place just outside the city. It was fantastic. Casual, homely, great service and the food looked delicious.

We ended up choosing four reasonably healthy tapas dishes of spicy Fijian chicken, garlic mushrooms, garlic prawns and spicy chorizo. The flavours in each dish turned out to be brilliant and, of course, I was very happy that Sonja had the same amount of garlic as I did!

I drank two glasses of red wine, and it tasted truly amazing. I realised how much I actually miss wine; its texture, the flavour. I even had a mild tingle from just two glasses. It was perfect.

Nutritionally I think we chose wisely. The chicken breasts were very tasty, as were the mushrooms and prawns. Except for a few extra fat grams in the chorizo (Spanish sausage) and some oil used to cook the other plates, I don't think I had too much excess fat. So while I technically did cheat, I did still show some restraint. All in all, we had a really nice, romantic, birthday meal.

If I'd given into temptation and splurged on chocolate cake, two bottles of wine, or a late night Aussie meat pie, I would really have been banging my head against the wall in disgust. But, I don't think I really did give into temptation. I took my girlfriend out for her birthday, and I think I owed her at least that for all her support. And, to be honest, I think I owed it to myself as well because it kind of acted as a reward of sorts for being so regimented throughout this past Caveman month.

So it's done, and I don't actually feel *too* badly about it. I'll get in a few extra jogging minutes this week, a few extra sit-ups and a few more arm curls so that, mentally and physically, the night out is counteracted.

Caveman Tip:

If you cheat, don't beat yourself up mentally. One day of deviance won't spoil forty days of training, so slap yourself on the wrist via a few extra minutes of training the next day, and move forward with the City Caveman Plan.

I guess I'll just have to wait and see what Annie has to say about this. And I will step up to the plate and accept the repercussions from her as they come; after all, being on the City Caveman Plan is all about accountability, right?

Annie says: *I knew the Austrian Devil would lead Mike astray eventually! I must be honest and admit I am a tad disappointed that he strayed from the Plan, but I also have to take into account that we are only human and not infallible. And I am glad it happened on Day 27 and not Day 7. At least he cheated for a good reason – his girlfriend's birthday – and since my birthday is on the same day, you could say I am a little understanding, especially since I didn't really give the City Caveman Plan much thought today either! Certainly, I would have wanted my Caveman boyfriend to stray from his Plan and take me out for my birthday dinner too!*

It is a good time to make the point that if you have chosen to undertake the 40-day City Caveman Plan, while it is a very important time in your life, do remember that the rest of the world still continues! Yes, nights out and a few parties will need to be sacrificed, but we still have weddings, birthday parties, and important business meetings where declaring 'sorry, I have to be a Caveman tonight' is perhaps not acceptable. Deviating from the City Caveman Plan will happen to us all at one point or another. But, in saying that, that does not give you free reign to do so whenever you want to. You still have a choice if you take a one-day break – you can jump in the deep end and eat and drink everything in sight, or you can tread lightly and enjoy just a slightly cheeky meal.

I consider Mike's night out as just a small Caveman stumble. He did choose wisely, and this will not radically impact his progress – tomorrow is a new day, and he can work off the Spanish food pretty easily, so no real harm done. So, at least Mike has proved that he is not a perfectionist and he is willing to be flexible for the girl he loves. But if he does it again, I will have him running the stairs ten times to work off a Spanish-style belly!

Remember, the City Caveman Plan is like slowly climbing a mountain over a 40-day period, and a night off is like taking one step backward. Keep that in mind, and it will ensure you do not go crazy on a night off and roll all the way back down the hill to the beginning.

Day 28. Temptation. It Never Goes Away

> *Opportunity may knock only once, but temptation leans on the doorbell.*
>
> – Author unknown

It's Sunday – my day off. I'm thinking back to my Friday night, when it was my mate's birthday dinner and drinks. It was probably the most difficult of all nights, and it's still in my head today. Even my memory is battling from it. We met in a cool little pub, and it was just one of those nights with a great vibe, good mates, lots of laughs, gossip and a good crowd out and about in Sydney – a perfect night for drinks and some great food.

And not just any food, but Mexican food. We had a table for twelve at a great place with piñatas hanging from the ceiling. The Mexican beer was flowing, the music was loud and the fruity tequila-based drinks were in abundance. And, of course, the menu contained every Mexican temptation you can think of: burritos, tacos, nachos, guacamole, spicy cheese dips and so on! I absolutely adore Mexican food.

And so there I was. The odd Caveman out. It felt like I was on the team but not allowed to actually leave the bench and play in the game. No drinks, and no food for me, thanks! Boo! And guess who was sitting nearby? The Scotsman. 'Hey, girly Mike, how does that Caveman water taste?' he teases, as he sips his margarita. He was tormenting me pretty good all night, actually. At one point he took a bite of his food and followed it up with some pseudo-orgasmic moaning and groaning. Jerk.

The upside of the night was that although I had to face all those tempting delights, I did receive a few compliments about how well I looked, with my skin and my fat loss. Those who hadn't seen me in a while did say they were quite impressed with my challenge and how well I looked physically as a result.

So, I do know that I am not immune to temptations or cravings, whether it is Day 1 or Day 26. My battle was Mexican-style tonight, and I won – again. Only two weeks to go! I don't mean to be a day-counter; I know that, just as when you're on holidays, you shouldn't count down the remaining days, but… only two weeks left! I almost can't believe it!

Caveman Tip:

Food temptations persist no matter what Caveman day it is. Keep battling, keep saying *no* and keep ticking the Caveman Contract boxes each night. You must win.

Annie's say: *As a fellow Mexican food lover, I sympathise with Mike's Friday night out for his mate's birthday. Sitting there watching people indulge while he sipped water would have been as hard as doing the stairs! I take my hat off to him. I had to do the same thing while I was dieting for my fitness competitions, so I know just how hard it is to keep saying 'no', especially when all you want to do is say 'bring* *it on!' But, like Mike did, keeping your eye on the finish line and keeping in mind why you are doing it all really can help you overcome temptations.*

I am very happy that Mike received recognition for the positive physical changes he's made so far. Compliments from friends and family are always encouraging and motivating to keep going.

At this point in time, I don't think I have any more advice for Mike regarding his food battles. He is pretty consistently facing those battles and winning, and now he's exchanged the bad habit of always saying 'yes' for the good habit of being able to make a choice and say 'no'. It really is all about storming the hard yards and continuing to check all the boxes so you can stick to the City Caveman Plan.

Day 29. Mental Ups & Downs

> *Life is a roller-coaster – you have your ups and downs, unless you fall off.*
>
> – Author unknown

It's Monday and it's officially Sonja's birthday! Early this morning we went for a walk across the Sydney Harbour Bridge with a breakfast planned at the end. What a lovely morning it was.

Watching Sonja eat her birthday French toast with berries, maple syrup and butter was not an easy task but at least I was distracted by the gorgeous Sydney harbour views. The setting was fantastic and our breakfast celebration was followed with a great little ferry ride home and some birthday kisses. It was a great start to what would turn out to be an up and down kind of day.

For some reason, I didn't feel excited to head to the gym today. Usually my Monday workouts are a buzz, but today my bounce was simply not there and, psychologically, I just wasn't into it. I'd received some disappointing news from a client who had decided not to proceed with a business idea I had, so that bummed me out a bit too.

Mentally and physically I was feeling pretty empty. It was quite frustrating to be unable to conjure up something to motivate me through, especially since I really did want to work off that Spanish meal from the weekend. I think maybe I'm just a bit physically drained today. Last Wednesday's Mount Everest and Friday's Stairway to Hell really took its toll on me, so maybe that was catching up with me today.

The first five minutes of my run felt like I was carrying a piano on my back. I just couldn't summon the energy I needed today. Physically, my legs did start to come back to me after a while but, mentally, I was just not into it. Still, I did my workout, feeling flat as I was, and hopefully tomorrow I will be in a better state of mind to deliver a better effort. In fact, I will decide to be; tomorrow I will give 110 per cent.

Caveman Tip:

Depressing days…well, they're part of life. Do your best to grind through them and give as close to 100 per cent effort as possible.

The day did get better when I saw some photos in Sonja's camera. There were old pictures in there, from when I visited Austria, from when Sonja visited Sydney during Christmas, and a couple of dinner pictures from Saturday's Spanish meal. So I actually got to see a comparison over time, of the physical changes that have occurred in me. And guess what? I can see them! The photos from Saturday night show me looking really, really slim and healthy and fit. I am really pleased that before I've even reached Day 30, I have achieved noticeable fat loss. For me, this means that from here on, I can fully concentrate on weights and improving my shape. Those photos were really exciting for me to see.

At the beginning of my journey, I told Annie that a major concern I had was my tendency to become complacent. So, if I found myself losing weight, the risk would be that I would potentially become a bit too comfortable with my progress and start treating myself to some cheeky meals and a few too many drinks. But, now that I am actually there and right in that very position, I actually don't feel like falling off the wagon. I feel like I am on the right track, and I am determined *not* to deviate.

The food I have been eating thus far has been tasty and plentiful and, while I miss a social wine or two, I do not miss the hangovers or the post-hangover workouts, nor do I miss the bloated tummy after a late night kebab. If my face looks thinner in photos and my usually-tight jeans have a surplus of room, then my shape *must* be improving. So let's hope the days of the pear-shaped body are finally over! With only eleven days to go, I am going to keep on cruising and enjoying this new lifestyle.

So, to bed for now, as I need some good rest for a big workout tomorrow. And a very happy birthday to Sonja and Annie!

Annie says: *It's my birthday! Yeah! I had an awesome day: lunch at my favourite restaurant, overlooking the Sydney Opera House, followed by afternoon tea with a girlfriend, and then another friend came over for dinner. I love being spoiled!*

I am happy that Mike still completed his workout and didn't have a dummy spit and go home early, even though he had a rough day, mentally. It is natural to have slow days, but the important thing is that you still go to the gym and complete your workout. Sometimes doing this can actually make you feel more energetic. And it is important to take your muscles through the motion; you are, after all, still building strength and burning calories even when you don't feel 100 per cent, so a workout at 70 per cent effort is better than nothing at all.

And finally, Mike actually saw the physical changes in himself via those photos! That's fantastic! I am glad he can see and enjoy his new look, after working so hard to get it. Often when people can't see their physical improvement in the mirror, they can see it in photos. There is no greater satisfaction for the mind than to see actual results occurring in the body. We put together our City Caveman Plan for the gym and the kitchen, and that Plan is finally definitely making a statement on Mike's body.

I will be equally excited for Mike to see himself in his 'after' photos after Day 40 – I just know he is going to fall in love with his new body! Of course, he better not become all cocky and arrogant, but I am confident the Caveman journey will keep him grounded and the same friendly person he was when he started this 40-day adventure.

Day 30. Caveman Sex and Nudity

> *Anybody who believes that the way to a man's heart is through his stomach flunked geography.*
>
> – Robert Byrne

Annie and I discussed my 'after' photos, which will be taken after Day 40. It'll be really interesting to look at the chubby photos side-by-side with the (hopefully) fit photos to see the difference. Annie has suggested (demanded) we take four pictures of me:

a wearing jeans and a t-shirt;
b posing in a workout stance with my workout gear on;
c topless in a pair of shorts; and
d nude.

Guess which one of the above I am shitting myself about? Nude. I don't know if I can go through with it, but we shall see. Let's just say a whole lot of coaxing and persuading will have to be done prior to that day. On Annie's website, she has some really cool photos with some half-naked, sexy pics. But hell, it's easy for her – she has a sexy body. For me? At least the photographer will get a good laugh that day. But, I trust Annie and her expertise in the area. So we made the photography appointment, and Annie confirms that she'll come along to help me with my poses on the day. As for whether *my boys* actually make an appearance, well that remains to be seen. It has been so long since I have felt comfortable with myself naked that to think about actually planning to take a nude photograph of myself, in front of other people, is a very daunting prospect!

But, the thought is enough motivation to get me to the gym!

I felt better today. My legs gave me a lot more than yesterday, and my run was pretty cruisey. I did not want to overdo it though, so I stayed at a pretty comfortable pace for the 40 minutes; it was a solid cardio workout. I'm happy to say that the 'squeeze' approach for my abs workout is still doing the trick, and while I would love those elusive six-pack abs at the end of my forty days, I do know that I have to be realistic. I am resigned to the fact that if I have a little chub left, then that is okay. I am not chasing perfection, after all, I am making a change to live a healthier lifestyle, and I will just keep telling myself that. If in the future I decide I do want that washboard stomach, then I can set it as a specific goal and focus on it then. But for now, a healthy lifestyle is first and foremost, as well as looking great in my jeans and a t-shirt.

Nudie photos are one thing but, at home, I have become a lot more confident being in the buff around Sonja. My body shape has improved and has given me a confidence I haven't had in a long, long time. I now look forward to when I can have naked nights on the couch, nice showers together and even a little naked cooking – it will open up a whole new world of fun! So, perhaps by the end of the forty days I'll have even more confidence, and perhaps I will even have enough to pose nude at that photography session. I guess time will tell.

So. Since we're on the cusp of the topic, let's just dive right in shall we? Sex. As I've already mentioned, throughout these past thirty days, my skin texture has improved, my non-hangover head has become clear, my eyes are healthier, and so on. And we touched on the fact that Sonja can benefit from the changes I am making to myself and, well, that is definitely true when it comes to the bedroom. The sex we have been having since I have become fitter and healthier and more confident in myself has been nothing short of outstanding. My stamina has increased, my recovery times are faster, I am stronger and more flexible and I can even honestly say that my orgasms are better.

Caveman Tip:

Better workouts in the gym and better sex in the bedroom – be aware and conscious of the benefits of the City Caveman Plan, as it will affect all parts of your healthy life.

So both Sonja and I appear to be enjoying the ever-increasing benefits from the City Caveman Plan. I am really happy to feel so much more confident in myself, and I will work towards increasing it enough to drop my strides in front of a photographer in ten days time. I really feel like I have found my Caveman groove now, because I am actually enjoying a new lifestyle, the ongoing challenges and my improved health.

Annie says: *Mike, I don't like you feeling embarrassed about your 'before' photo, because that's no longer the person I see before me. In fact, I want you to keep that picture on hand to serve as a reminder of what you used to look like and what you should never revert to being. Using this type of scare tactic might seem harsh, but I am confident that the 'before' and 'after' comparison will be a real trophy for you, to illustrate exactly how far you have come on this journey.*

As for not having a six-pack – it's only Day 30! There are still ten days to go and I am betting that by Day 40 (and just in time for the photo shoot) you will have a six-pack! I want you to just keep on forging ahead with 'squeeze' workouts, keep eating our low-fat meals and, together, this combination will show results! Also remember that sometimes muscle definition is best seen from a distance, so try not to judge too harshly from what you see in the bathroom mirror.

Now, the sex. Isn't Sonja lucky? Mike is becoming a better lover in the bedroom! I can tell you, from experience, that men who work out do make better lovers. Feeling good about your body increases your sense of touch and feel, your confidence, as well as your sex drive. So intimacy, naturally, becomes better too.

These days there are a million ads on the radio and in your email inbox which promote drugs to combat erectile dysfunction. In my earlier days as a pharmaceutical sales rep, I actually did promote a drug for erectile dysfunction, so I do know a lot about those drugs. One thing that isn't common knowledge, however, is that the first line treatment for the condition is actually exercise and a low fat diet. This is because the major cause of erectile dysfunction is poor health and high blood pressure.

Interestingly, I also promoted drugs to treat type 2 diabetes and hypertension and the first line treatment for both of those conditions is also exercise and a low fat diet. Unfortunately, though, people seek medicine rather than looking at their own actions to see how they can improve their health. So what happens when the medicines don't do the trick? Potentially you could be facing operations or life-long diseases – yet all the while, a tried and tested cure that doesn't cost the earth is right in front of you. It's called living a healthy life!

14

City Caveman Days 31 to 40 – *Understanding Change*

Day 31. New Adventures

> *Never be afraid to try something new. Remember, amateurs built the ark. Professionals built the Titanic.*
>
> – Author unknown

Annie sent me an email this morning that read:

> *Hey, you said your legs were feeling a little off in the last few days. Skip your regular run today and get yourself into an indoor cycling class. You will enjoy it.*

Wow, it had been years since I was in a cycle class, but I did enjoy doing them. The classes are usually held in a darkish room with the instructor's bike up on a stage facing out to the class. The class participants are then perched on the 50 or so bikes that all face toward the stage. The instructor usually plays loud, groovy music and tells participants to increase or decrease the friction on the wheel and to pedal faster or slower, all the while creating a really unique and effective resistance training class.

Before the start of my class, I did a little stretching and ran a kilometre or so to warm up. I noticed that people were starting to gather outside the cycle studio so I went over to make sure I would be able to get a bike too. At that moment the people from the class that had just finished started to pour out of the room and, much to my horror, they all had expressions of 'holy shit, I am exhausted' on their faces, and they all looked like they had just gone swimming from the volume of sweat that was soaked into their clothes and dripping on the floor around them. Was it seriously that hard a class? I didn't recall that part of the class from my former indoor cycling days!

I wanted to choose a bike in the middle of the room, so I didn't look like teacher's pet in the front row, but so I also wouldn't look like I had something to hide by hanging in the back row.

As it happened though, I got bustled into the room and ended up in the second row which I thought would be fine; however, no one sat in front of me so I was right in the firing line of the instructor. Gulp. The teacher was just as you would expect: ultra-fit with no body fat, and legs as thick as Sequoia tree trunks. After wrestling with my bike to make sure the configuration fit my size and riding style, we were off. The music was absolutely pumping. It definitely wasn't the sort of music I'd choose to listen to, but the beat was so strong it helped to set my pedalling pace.

The class was a good test on the legs. Some songs were slower with a heavy bass beat and, during those tracks, we increased the friction on the wheel so our pedalling was slower. Other tracks were faster, so we eased up on the wheel tension and sprinted, using really fast pedal revolutions. Sometimes we stood up to pedal, sometimes we sat down and sometimes we hovered just over the top of our seats using maximum friction, which really worked the hamstrings and bum. It was a really good legs workout, and I was faring pretty well.

I know it is an old joke, but honestly, if we can send a man to the moon almost forty years ago, why isn't there a bike seat that doesn't smash my testicles? The pain is not fun and, with drinking so much water prior to my workout, I was ready for a toilet break before the first half of the class was over!

All in all, my reunion with the cycle class was challenging. Forty-five minutes on a bike with sprints and uphill climbs is a good workout, and when I jumped off the bike, I realised exactly how great: my legs wouldn't move as fast as I'd have liked them to. The time really did fly during that class. I guess because you don't have time to think about it when you're being told to do this, do that, visualise this, picture that. It was only when I left the room that I realised how much I'd been sweating. I looked just like those people I'd seen earlier. I was tired, but it felt great.

Caveman Tip:

Don't be afraid to mix up your workouts. Physically and mentally you will appreciate the variety. Just keep moving!

The change in my workout was excellent. My knees needed an altered pace, and I was able to give my body just as vigorous a workout as normal but in a different, exciting forum.

Annie says: *As Mike's trainer, I could tell from his writing and his thoughts that his body was in need of a change. This is a good thing. It is a really good idea to mix up your training every once in a while and do something new. That way, your muscles do not get used to one thing or one type of movement, and they are more likely to get stronger and you are more likely to improve your fitness and burn more calories. Indoor cycling classes certainly provide a hard workout in a unique and motivating environment, so they can be enjoyable but challenging as well.*

So, as you are going through the City Caveman Plan and you think 'I just need a break from my normal cardio workout', this is the perfect way to add some variety. Take the opportunity as one where you can try what you might have been intrigued but too scared to have a go at. Always wanted to experience a cycling class? Give it a go! Thought about swimming a few laps in the pool? Do it! Intrigued to know what the stair challenge feels like? Have a go! The City Caveman Plan is not set in stone. It is a great guide to providing a balanced cardiovascular and weights program that is achievable for everyone. But when you mentally or physically need a change from the norm, experiment a little and find what workout styles suit you. Then do them! Your body and your mind will thank you in the short and longer term for making small changes while you continue on the overall Plan.

Day 32. New Body, New Jeans

> *Nobody's a natural. You work hard to get good and then work hard to get better.*
>
> – Paul Coffey

I am what one might call *klutzy-coordinated*. I say that because I am pretty good with my hand-eye coordination, such as being on the golf course or the basketball court, but I can also be a total klutz. For example, at dinner: it could be the first bite or it could be the last bite, but on most occasions, I will spill something on my shirt when I eat. It's a Jarosky trait that I inherited from Dad. Away from the dinner table, I usually fare a little better in the klutz stakes, but that was until today.

I went to a gym that is different to my usual one. This one has a lot of ultra-fit guys and high-society women strutting around. I thought I would start my warm up with some rope-jumping and, having become pretty adept at it over the past thirty days I felt quite confident about the left-leg-only, right-leg-only, double-jumps routines that I'd concocted. (You name it, and I can do it with the speed of a wanna-be boxer!)

So this morning I started my skipping. 1-2-3-4-5-6-7…I started moving faster, then faster… 8-9-10…whip, snap, whip, snap and 'OW SHIT!'

I'd managed to pick up a pretty decent pace, but the rope caught on the carpet (I usually do it on the wooden studio floor), and then proceeded to whip me in the chest like a damn lasso. And the worst bit? The rope was made of leather, so it hurt like hell. I lifted up my shirt to see a thick, long, red welt appearing down my chest. A war wound proclaiming victory over another Caveman battle. Well, sort of.

During my abs workout, I started thinking of how far I had come. Three weeks ago, doing sit-ups, push-ups, or bicep curls made me wince in pain, complain to Sonja, or call Annie looking for sympathy. But now, I've learned how to accept that pain, and so much so that I have turned the corner where I honestly don't think I could describe it as pain. Nowadays, it's simply the feeling of my muscles working and changing.

After my workout, I thought I would do a hint of shopping to take advantage of the end-of-financial-year sales. The pair of jeans that I wear quite often has started to hang a little too much off my hips, so I thought I could pick up a new pair and a t-shirt or two.

Now, normally I'd stock up on jeans from home, where Levi's are a steal at around $30, but today I ended up in some swanky designer boutique, where I discovered an amazing looking pair of jeans.

The salesgirl asked me my size. I had no idea.

I couldn't help but giggle a bit, when she suggested I try on a pair of size 32s, and I was astounded to find that when I tried them on they were too big.

She then told me that since they did not carry a size 31, I should try the 30. Size 30? I could barely believe my ears. The last time I was wearing size 30 was when I was 17 years old and in third year at high school. So you can imagine my astonishment when I came out of the dressing room and the size 30s fitted my waist perfectly.

'Ah yes, now those are perfect for you. They show off your nice bum,' the girl said. (Was she flirting with me? Or just spilling sales-girl crap so I would pay $229 for these jeans?).

'Yeah, these are definitely the nicest jeans I have ever worn. They are surprisingly comfy in the waist, but they are bit tight through the legs and, pardon my French, but the midsection here is so tight that you can nearly see if I'm circumcised.'

'Ha, ha,' she laughed (a little nervously?), 'but that *is* the style, and they do look good.'

'Okay, well let me have a think about it. Thanks so much,' I said.

Size 30. I couldn't get over it. I was wearing a size 36 waist just a little over a month ago, which means I've dropped six sizes without even noticing.

I understand now why people get so overjoyed about dropping dress or clothing sizes when they lose weight; it feels fantastic. I really debated over the purchase of those jeans, even to the point where I got into an SMS debate with my brother in

Chicago. He told me to buy them because I deserved them. But, in the end I just couldn't do it. The upside was that I was on such a high knowing how drastically my waist size had decreased that I didn't want to jeopardise the high with potential buyer's remorse.

All the hard work, all the good eating has finally paid off.

Size 30? Woohoooooooooooo!

Caveman Tip:

Be it Day 20 or Day 32, when you reach your ideal weight, waist size, dress size, run time, or whatever…stay committed and see out the City Caveman Plan all the way to Day 40.

Annie says: *We are all prone to the embarrassing gym mishaps, from falling off a moving treadmill to dropping weights that are too heavy to press. These things happen, and sporting the war wounds from a gym injury shows not only that Mike is a trooper, but it's also a rite of passage when you are travelling from fat to fit.*

Concerning the pain of his workouts, I am glad that Mike's pain has transformed into the pleasure of feeling his muscles getting a good workout. I see 'workout pain' in three stages; unfortunately, too many people give up during the first stage, unaware of the second stage, which is much more pleasant and tolerable. The third stage, which is where I'm at, is where I do not feel like I have had a good weights workout unless I have felt my muscles experiencing absolute failure on the last set. Once you get to that stage, you never have to worry about putting on weight because by then, fitness becomes a passion and a lifestyle and so, more often than not, you have to be dragged out of the gym rather than to it.

The beauty is that as you move from one stage to the next, 'pain' as initially felt transforms itself from tolerable to pleasurable.

I am also very impressed to see Mike back into the size 30 jeans. And salesladies telling him he has a hot arse? Nice one! Let's make sure his head does not get too big, or his weight could go up again!

Mike's confidence and self-esteem are blossoming as he starts reaping the positive results of his hard work in the gym and from his healthy diet. Mike deserves to feel proud of his accomplishments and the pleasure that he, and all of us, can get from looking and feeling great. It will ensure that we continue along with our healthy habits in the days, months and years to come.

Day 33. Health versus Beauty

> *If I had been around when Rubens was painting, I would have been revered as a fabulous model. Kate Moss? Well, she would have been the paintbrush.*
>
> – Dawn French

With the weather in Sydney taking a turn for the worse, an outdoor run with Annie was not possible – at least this saves me a potential torturous run up Mount Holy Shit. So, off to the gym I went, solo.

I pushed myself pretty hard on the treadmill today, knowing that, had I been with Annie, she would have been giving me a flogging up that hill. Also, for some reason, it feels good to be huffing and puffing inside the gym when it is pouring down outside.

While in the zone, my mind started to wander back to a few nights ago when I was watching *Australia's Next Top Model*. What drew me into watching the show was that the eventual winner was a girl who is 185cm and weighs 58kgs.

Now let's be honest. Most super skinny models with those measurements cannot swim laps, they cannot run for ten minutes at a decent pace and they do not eat balanced meals. They are the epitome of unhealthy. So, I will have to agree with an interviewee on the news that said something to the effect of, 'The winner could certainly be admitted to hospital at that weight.'

My point is obvious. Television shows like *Australia's Next Top Model* and the fashion/magazine/beauty industries have all become entirely disassociated with the fact that there is a difference between *health* and *beauty*.

Caveman Tip:

The fashion industry and Hollywood will always chase the obscure, the unobtainable, the *beautiful*. But what will always be trendy, in style and truly beautiful is a healthy mind and a healthy body.

For some reason, we are all brainwashed into thinking that skinny is beautiful. Yet the truth is that not only is skinny *not* necessarily beautiful, but it can also be downright dangerous. In fact, last year, two Uruguayan sisters, who were both high profile models, died of anorexia. The industry started to take a look at itself, but then Australia goes and selects another skeletal girl as its top model.

It really saddens me how influential television and magazines affect people's perceptions of what is desirable, because often what is deemed *beautiful* is, in fact, *unhealthy*.

Annie says: *Mike is so right; people who are too skinny are just as unhealthy as those who are obese. Models and actresses today have millions of young girls aspiring to be exactly like them, but like Mike said, most of those ultra-skinny types cannot swim, run, hike, bike or lead any type of consistently active lifestyle.*

I, like many I hope, do not find ultra-skinny, waif-like women attractive. I actually feel a bit sorry for them because I wonder about what they deny themselves in order to retain that body shape. They don't get to enjoy nice food; they can't indulge in a nice hike on a sunny day. Instead, they might be taking drugs and living on rice crackers, denying everything that life has on offer just so they can be someone's coat hanger for a while. The bottom line is that clothes designers like tall skinny women to show off their clothes because the garments hang off them well (just like a moving coat hanger) and so they sell more!

Body size can be a reflection of what society wants to see. For example, if publishers sell more magazines when they have skinny models in them, then they will keep putting those people in their pages. We should not be embracing diets to achieve an emaciated Hollywood frame. Instead, my attitude towards body image and size is reflected in the design of the City Caveman Plan. It is all about leading a balanced, active life and making a change so that you can feel good about your body and your mind for the long haul. Now THAT is healthy, fashionable and beautiful.

Day 34. From drinking to groceries – we all have options

> *I don't consider fat a disease. I mean, c'mon, who had the gun to my head? Nobody. What gene in my body says I have to eat four cakes instead of two? It's a choice.*
>
> – Kirstie Alley

Last night's party was another reminder of how difficult it is to socialise without alcohol. If I were to start my challenge all over again, I would probably have avoided a few more of those types of nights, because it really is difficult.

This month is officially birthday month for the masses! I have about eight friends who have birthdays and, to top it off, I have my own! Last night another four combined birthday parties were being held at a swanky city bar. Again, it was one of those nights where three hundred people are dancing to funky music, plenty of drinks are flowing and everyone is really into it – except, of course, Caveman Mike.

Champagne, vodka martinis, Coronas, they're all breezing right by me. Loud music, girls in sexy dresses, drunken folks laughing hysterically…I felt so out of place and like I just didn't belong.

I still have a way to go regarding my elimination of alcohol. I have been so good about not drinking over these five weeks, but I still feel this angst when I socialise, as if I'm being left out of something fantastic if I'm not drinking. Physically, I have succeeded in doing it, but psychologically I know I am not there yet.

On a positive note though, quite a few people came up to me and said, 'Wow, Mike, you look great.' Compliments were quite forthcoming, which kind of helped ease the pain of feeling so isolated.

Thankfully, I stayed true to the City Caveman Plan, and although this was a damn good party, it was a party like any other that will be available to me after the 40-day Plan is completed, so I shall wait it out and have drinks then.

Now that I think about it, perhaps my frustration doesn't actually stem from the lack of drinking so much, but maybe it's more to do with the comments that come with being a non-drinker. I don't mind a bit of ball-busting, and I can give it out as much as anybody, but last night a few people were dishing it out a little heavier than I'd have liked. Maybe I was being overly sensitive, but it bugged me when they would say things like, 'Ah, we'll see the old Mike come back to us next week,' or, 'Don't worry Sonja, he will be back with us and legless in seven days.'

I don't know. It kind of hurts to think that now I'm considered the nerd of the group when, deep down, I'm actually feeling physically and mentally in the best shape of my life.

It's like there's this tug-of-war inside me, trying to work out how to do the right things for my mind and body in order to make a positive change, while also keeping good with my mates who just want me to get drunk and party hard like we used to.

Realising that my mates don't appreciate the life change that I am trying to achieve also kind of sucks. This has been one of the hardest battles I've faced in my thirty-four days as a Caveman. I equate it to being a student at university; if you were the guy who tried to get a bit of studying done when everybody else was having some sneaky beers on a Tuesday afternoon, you were considered an outcast. Yet the only reason you were looked down upon was because your studying made the others feel guilty about doing something they knew they should also be doing.

Caveman Tip:

Some friends will embrace your desire to change; others will disapprove of your positive strides. Ignore the negative, and welcome the positive.

The rain continued today. Umbrellas were useless as anything put into the wind was whisked away, so it was a quick train ride to Bondi and off to the mall gym for a good Saturday run. After my run and some unsuccessful shoe shopping, we had grocery shopping to do. Fruit, bok choy, chicken and a few other healthy goodies were on the menu. Luckily Sonja was too tired and hung over to put some Caveman cheating items in the trolley, so I was able to sneak only the healthiest of items home. But, while we were walking down the potato chip aisle seeking out rice crackers, I couldn't help but pick up a packet of crisps for the sole purpose of checking the nutrient contents. I was startled to find that in a mid-sized packet of crisps there are 35 grams of fat, which is more than the City Caveman Plan is allowing me for a whole day!

The City Caveman Plan is all about my new body, my new lifestyle and my new approach to shopping at the grocery store. The least I can do in the future is to take a look at the labels of things I want to consume. It's all about a little extra time and thought and being educated enough to make informed decisions. While my 30+ days in the City Caveman Plan has not turned me into a certified nutritionist, it has shown me some pretty good options in order to maintain a lower fat, lower sodium and lower sugar diet without giving away all the taste. I love my newfound *power to choose*, even if it does take a little more planning and creativity to achieve.

Annie says*: I can empathise with Mike's presence at the party and not being able to drink. I went through it when competing in fitness competitions and also while pregnant (which, of course, was NINE months, not a mere forty days!). In both circumstances I felt like the odd one out and that I was missing out on some fun. But, interestingly, people were more tolerant of my teetotalling lifestyle when I was doing it due to my pregnancy, rather than for my own health during fitness competitions. So what does that say? That it is okay to avoid toxins in a bid to protect your unborn child, but it is not okay to do it for yourself?*

There is also an element of jealousy when you start looking fit and healthy. People can be a little envious of 'the new you' and want to bring you back to their level. And when someone is doing something wrong, they like others to do it too so, as Mike said, they do not feel so guilty about it.

Let's face it: binge drinking is wrong for so many reasons, so I'm glad that they weren't able to sway Mike to join them in their toxic consumption. I promise you, Mike, that you will look and feel better for having restrained yourself, yet again, at another Sydney party.

Developing Mike's approach to grocery shopping provides a reference point to at least train your brain to think 'Is there a healthier option than this?' each time you are buying food. Think of what you have, and just give a split second's thought to 'Could I go healthier?' And over time you will condition yourself so that you will not even see the unhealthy choices – you will go right to the lower fat, healthier item. It is then that you will know you have truly made the Caveman change.

Day 35. A Health Revolution

It is health that is real wealth and not pieces of gold and silver.

– Gandhi

Today was a day of deep-thought for me.

I want to gain a better grasp of what is most important in my life, and I think that it is my health.

We are all so focused on the material things. More money, more toys, more stuff, more food, more wealth, more, more, more. Our cars are bigger than ever, and our waistlines are following the auto-makers' lead. Sometimes I wonder: when is enough going to be enough? Why is *more stuff* and *bigger things* so appealing to so many? When will we stop wanting more – and not only *more*, but more than the other guy?

It's all bullshit really, isn't it? I want a revolutionary shift in thinking to take place, so that there is no more 'I want more because more is better' mentality. And in its place I want people to start asking themselves: Do I really need all this stuff? And: Do I really need to consume more?

I'm not having my own *Jerry Maguire* moment, but it just seems that today our culture is so much about 'want, want, want' and 'more, more, more' that we have lost focus on what is actually the most important thing of all – our health.

On the footpath is a fit, smiling, healthy, 65-year-old couple holding hands going for a walk, and on the street right next to them is an overweight millionaire driving a red Ferrari. Which of those two would people admire most often? The Ferrari, of course. This is because, too often, we admire *wealth* instead of *health*.

So where is the documentary about our own inability to care for ourselves, highlighting the deathly trend of obesity, diabetes and heart issues? For the first time in human civilisation, children today will die at a younger age than the preceding generation. *We are feeding ourselves to death with too much sugar, too much fat and too much processed shit*. This is society's true demon and we're losing the battle. It's not the *next* big story – it's yesterday's, today's and tomorrow's front page news. Where is Michael Moore when we need him? Eating.

The environment is all you hear about on the news and in magazines, but I sometimes think we are a bit ahead of ourselves in this regard. How can we expect ourselves, as a society, to care about the environment when the statistical majority cannot properly take care of themselves? I really doubt you'd find a guy who just downed two value meals with an apple pie and a two-litre fizzy drink ensuring he throws his trash into the proper recycle bins! It needs to start with us, and us alone. Let's stop polluting our bodies and our minds (the inside) with so much junk food and junk drink, and then we will be able to transfer our concern to the environment (the outside).

Caveman Tip:

Fix yourself first, and you will be better equipped to fix the environment.

When you think about it, the environment and our bodies are the same. We both suffer from an overdose of too many chemicals and now we are both sick and endangered. I do think it's about respect, and respecting our bodies should be our number one priority.

***Annie says**: Mike and I spoke about this over our first lunch together, and I couldn't agree more. Respecting our bodies and our minds is a direct parallel to how we respect our environment, and a health revolution can only start one person at a time – with YOU. Then that revolution can spread, to your partner and on to your children. A health revolution is infectious but it's an infection that our society is in need of.*

Scientists don't believe it's too late to fix the environment, and I don't believe it's ever too late to fix our health. But, we must take the TIME TO LEARN and expend the ENERGY TO CHANGE in order to make both of these things happen.

Day 36. My Body has Changed

> *Nothing builds self-esteem and self-confidence like accomplishment.*
>
> – Thomas Carlyle

I can now say with certainty that I have changed.

My skin is clear.
My eyes look fresh.
My time on the toilet is healthy.
My run times have improved immensely.
The joints in my legs and whole body feel better.
I eat healthy breakfasts filled with energy.
At night I am 'fit tired' rather than 'fat/bloated tired'.
I have had NO hangovers.
I do not snack on shit food.
My strength has improved.
My cardiovascular condition has improved.
My mind/body confidence has increased.

But the best part? I feel fucking great! It is difficult to express how good it feels to be slim and fit. That 'bounce' I spoke about from the treadmill has penetrated into every part of my life now; mornings are no longer a struggle, and I have energy throughout every part of the day. Being a City Caveman has affected my mind and body, as well as my relationships and all other aspects within my life in a very positive way.

I feel so grateful to have been able to create and take on the City Caveman Plan because the improvements in my mental health from becoming so physically transformed are amazing.

We all have a choice, and we all face battles regarding our health but from this day on, I will be so happy to continue the fight. For I am hooked. I am choosing a slim, fit and healthy lifestyle forever.

In making this choice and achieving my plan of change, now I am at the point where I can set some physical goals for myself that I would not have been able to get near prior to the City Caveman Plan.

So what are my plans? The six-pack abs or the bulging guns for arms? I know that if wanted those things I could work out a plan to get me there; however, for now I just want to maintain my current state of health and happiness, and I think by creating some simple yet demanding physical goals, I will be able to do so.

For example, today I just signed up for the City to Surf run on the 12th of August. It is a pretty tough 14-kilometre run with uphill and downhill sections. Running it a few years back, I remember stopping in a pub to do a shot of Southern Comfort to ease my hangover. What a runner, eh? Well, in two months, I will challenge myself with this run again, and my goal is to finish around the 70-minute mark, which would qualify me to run in the lead group the following year. I think this would be a demanding yet achievable challenge that will test my fitness and running ability. It's great knowing that I am now in a condition to be able to take on a whole host of physical challenges that I couldn't have done before.

Caveman Tip:

When you change for the good, a new life develops – embrace this new life and take on new challenges.

These days, good, hard, tiring workouts have become a part of my day, just as reliably as healthy breakfasts have. My body and my mind expect it, and I hate to use the word habit, because thinking of workouts as a habit isn't necessarily positive, but my workouts have become great therapy in my pursuit to become fit and healthy.

I know that some of my friends are expecting me to celebrate the completion of the City Caveman Plan this weekend by going and sitting in a pub to play catch-up for forty days of non-drinking; however, they are misled. Sure, I will celebrate on Friday with a couple of glasses of wine, but there will be no return to the eight-martinis-with-a-beef-and-cheese-kebab-chaser lifestyle. I still plan to have a great Saturday workout, continue to eat healthy meals and sleep in with the Austrian Devil. I should probably tell my mates now that this *changed life* is actually a *change for life*.

Annie says: *Visual reminders are very powerful in helping us achieve what we want. I have a vision board that I look at every day. One side has pictures of my top five goals on it; the other side has pictures of what I am grateful for in my life right now. I would encourage you to create your own vision board. It not only gives you direction for the future, but it also keeps you in touch with how lucky you are and how good your life is in the present.*

I am really pleased that Mike has achieved all those physical benefits from following the plan and ticking the boxes on a daily basis. I have seen him transform before my very eyes, and I am really impressed with his willpower and drive to stick to the plan, even though at times it was hard. And he describes the change as not just physical but psychological as well. He not only looks fit and healthy but also has a confidence and sense of wellbeing about him that he did not have before.

I think many people are in denial about their poor state of health. Mike is just the opposite as he has not yet accepted that he has the body and the abs he always wanted. I cannot wait for him to realise it when he sees his photos.

Goals such as running the City to Surf in 70 minutes are positive and achievable. I am glad he is looking to the future with new fitness goals, rather than thinking about readopting his old life.

Now, please let me clarify something: there is nothing wrong with thinking that workouts are habitual! Good habits that become permanent parts of your lifestyle are worth celebrating! Workouts certainly are a habit for Mike now, which is great, but if he needs to call them 'great therapy' instead, then no problems; whatever works for him!

I am and will be a fitness fanatic for the rest of my life; and I think Mike will be too.

Day 37. The Magical Fat Loss Cure

> *Magic is believing in yourself, if you can do that, you can make anything happen.*
>
> – Johann Wolfgang von Goethe

On my way home tonight, I stopped to buy some toothpaste and shampoo, and at the checkout I snooped a little bit and noticed the chap in front of me buying a new, over-the-counter medication that works to prevent the absorption of some of the fat from food. I found online that this drug is marketed under different names in different countries and the parent company's website makes reference to the side effects, suggesting, 'You may feel an urgent need to go to the bathroom. Until you have a sense of any treatment effects, it's probably a smart idea to wear dark pants, and bring a change of clothes with you to work.'

Great. So scientists have now created a drug that attempts to get you slim at the expense of crapping in your pants on a daily basis? Is this what obtaining health has come to?

It's a shame…the hope, the want, the wish for so many people: The Magical Fat Pill.

We could become the ultimate, master-consumers…eating, eating and more eating along with a few too many beers, with no remorse and no care. We would still be thin at the drop of the daily fat pill. The major pharmaceutical companies must be continuing to work 24/7 to try and find that magical cure for hundreds of millions of us…that one pill to make us all slim and sexy.

Would it really make us healthier? People could eat a greasy breakfast, down a fast-food lunch and a pizza at dinner, then take a bedtime pill and shed those fat grams and still be thin. Good on the outside, but what about the inside? All those chemicals, all that junk – it would all still pass through our bodies. So our organs, our teeth, our eyes and our health would still be close to death. We would be walking corpses – thin ones.

Science plays a fantastic role in sending man to space, but when some folks will be holidaying in space in the next 10 years, some of us will still put a higher value on a holiday which entails a simple three-hour car ride, a beach hut and a lovely view to a sunset on the beach. I am in that group – the group that loves simplicity. Complex scientific trends are fantastic and interesting, but they are not for everybody. And as workouts and wacky diet pills move into this futuristic realm, I am so glad I have been able to make a change while bucking these trends.

Caveman Tip:

Weight loss will never be about the 'trendy' or the 'magical'. It will always be *simple* – healthy eating and efficient workouts.

I even discussed some of this with the friendly photographer who is shooting the 'after' photos, and he was interested to know if the City Caveman Plan would work for a soon-to-be 60-year-old. I do not even need to have Annie's professional background to answer this, because that answer is 'YES'. Healthy eating, plenty of water and effective yet simple workouts will work for EVERYBODY! And if running is not your thing, then you just have to choose something you really enjoy doing, like weights, cycling (indoors or outdoors), yoga, Pilates, walking, rowing, boxing, swimming, dancing – there is no limit!

Annie says: *Mike's positive changes are inspiring other people to take on the City Caveman Plan. And that is exactly what we want to happen. We want to help as many people as possible to feel fit and healthy. And now that I have seen Mike emerge as a beautiful butterfly after thirty-seven days on the plan, I am even more motivated to help spread the health message to as many people as I can. Eating well and performing efficient workouts isn't just for guys and, although our Caveman tag sounds blokey, this Plan is for men, women, the young, and (politely speaking) the old.*

For those who are waiting for the magical fat pill, I urge you to take on the City Caveman Plan in the meantime – you'll be so much better off for it.

Day 38. HOT Yoga

I tried yoga once but took off for the mall halfway through class, as I had a sudden craving for a soft pretzel and world peace.

– Terri Guillemets

When it is 40 degrees outside, you can normally find me doing anything to dodge the heat. However, tonight I exercised in it.

Annie had said, 'Hey Mike, let's mix it up again and get you to a Bikram yoga class.'

Bikram yoga? What's Bikram yoga?

Definition of Bikram yoga: a series of 26 postures conducted over 90 minutes, beginning with a breathing exercise to warm up, progressing through 24 asanas (postures) and finishing with a toxin-eliminating breathing posture. This series of postures was scientifically designed to systematically work through the entire body.[vii]

For simplicity, below is my definition:

Caveman Mike's Definition of Bikram yoga: Yoga that you do in a fucking hot, hot, hot room.

I arrived pretty early to fill out some paperwork. I signed some form that eliminated their liability in case I melted, left my boots at the front of the studio and headed upstairs to the men's change room where one chap was getting ready.

'Excuse me,' I said. 'Where do I leave my bag so that it does not get stolen?'

'Ha ha. Nothing gets taken here. Just leave it in the corner and it will be there when you get out 90 minutes later,' the guy replied.

Maybe this is a non-issue, but for me, this 'leave your bag wherever' feature is pretty much a highlight for me, because for years I have been staring at annoying gym signs that read: Please safeguard your valuables as management is not

vii Bikram's Yoga College of India, 2008, 'Bikram's Yoga', <http://www.bikram.com.au/bikram_yoga.htm>.

responsible for stolen items. Seriously – the nerve of these gyms to remove themselves from liability when your favourite watch, wallet, or phone go missing? It just doesn't seem fair.

So, my first thought about yoga was that I loved the Buddhist style of 'We are here to relax, exercise, meet and enjoy.' The spiritual overtone of the place was pretty cool.

I entered the room, and I immediately made mistake number one, which is…do not get overly excited about Bikram yoga.

Playing basketball? Lifting weights? Going for a big run? Get yourself excited, get pumped up and get ready! But with yoga? Change gears, and be very, very low key. The tone of the studio is quiet and calm. Nobody talks, nobody warms up. In fact most were laying down on their backs with their legs out straight and their palms facing upwards. Add 40 degrees worth of heat to the image, and welcome to Bikram yoga.

In my view, I could see the two vents that were pumping out the air, so I knew to steer clear of them. The room was so hot. I lay out my yoga mat and towel in the back corner of the room, and lay down like the others, but with my feet facing the front of the room. I was fidgeting with my towel a bit, when I noticed a friendly girl walking my way, looking as if she was about to tell me something.

Enter, mistake number two. She said:

It is considered rude to have the soles of your feet facing forward, so you should just lay down the other way, palms up, head back, and relax a bit until we get started.

Oops.

Soon enough, the instructor came in and we began the class. Well, they began. I was met with mistake number three.

The back of the room in yoga does not mean you are out of the instructor's sight or mind.

Apparently yoga is not like a cycling class where the instructor is stationary at the front for the whole time. In Bikram yoga the teacher weaves around the class members to help them make sure their poses are done correctly and safely. There are two types of yoga attendees: the regulars, and the brand new formerly chubby chaps giving it their first try.

I had been told that Bikram yoga has the same poses and positions no matter where you practice it throughout the world. At times I felt like a snake charmer, or maybe more like the snake itself, wiggling and contorting my body into odd positions (26, to be exact). What I learned from this session was that Bikram yoga is a true test of breathing, flexibility, core strength and concentration.

If you do not breathe properly, you will pass out. If you are not flexible, yoga positions are impossible. If you do not have core strength, you will not have the stability to stop yourself from falling over. And if you do not concentrate 100 per cent, well, you might as well not even show up.

Concentration is key, and it was definitely the highlight of the night. Bikram is an escape from the world. Your mind is 100 per cent focused on finding and maintaining an out-of-this-world pose. There are no mobile phones, there is no chatting and there are no windows to view the outsiders. It is truly an experience of escapism.

And not only are the positions very, very difficult to maintain, but coming out of them is no easy task either. You do not just pop out of a Bikram pose. You slowly come out of it in the same mode you went into it.

Amazingly, I made it through the full 90 minutes. Now, I don't think they'll be putting a plaque up on the wall dedicated to my wonderful performance, but I gave it a try and, even though there were many poses I couldn't do, I left there feeling like I'd had a great workout and experienced something really new and different to anything else I'd experienced during the Caveman journey.

Over the years, my brother, among other friends in the States, had recommended Bikram yoga to me, and now that I had experienced it first-hand, their description of what it felt like post-class, was spot on. They'd told me, 'You will leave yoga in an altered and euphoric state.' It really is hard to describe; it could be the blood flow, it could be the strange poses, or it could be the need for fluids and recovery, but you truly feel different. It is a really cool workout, and it is very effective in moving your mind and body into a different, yet unique space.

I have a long way to go before I 'master' Bikram, but it was great for me to give another effective form of exercise a try, even if I did stumble my way through a lot of it.

Caveman Tip:

Try something outside of your *laziness zone*…and fitness and health will soon become part of your *comfort zone*.

Once I got home, I had to get my sweat-drenched clothes off and jump into the shower. It was then that I noticed mistake number four – I'd left my new boots which were less than a week old at the yoga entrance. Damn!

Annie says: *Bikram yoga is such an amazing, unique experience. I remember doing my one and only class several years ago for an article I wrote about group fitness classes to try. And my experience was much like Mike's; I loved the heat and I also left feeling euphoric.*

When trying any new exercise that differs from what you're used to, it is really important to remember to stretch afterwards so you do not tighten up the next day. The beauty of yoga is that doing a class every now and then ensures that you are maintaining and improving your flexibility.

I was confident that Mike's yoga session would challenge some muscles he may have been missing out on with the weights and running. And this is why cross-training is so effective: it ensures your whole body gets a full workout.

Also, it makes life more fun and interesting; after all, it is crazy to expect an individual to think that they will stare at the same treadmill in the same gym and perform the same exercises forever, without getting bored.

As we know and as we've seen, using a variety of physical and mental challenges can have profound effects on your health.

The countdown continues for my Bikram Caveman, as only two days in the Cave remain!

Day 39. Bye Bye Cravings

Discipline is the bridge between goals and accomplishments.

– Jim Rohn

It has taken some time, and I am not exactly sure when it happened. Last week? Just today? But through practice, I have become disciplined, and I believe I have finally won the biggest battle of them all – the food battle.

I did my usual walk to the gym today, passing by the smell of the doughnut shop, chicken schnitzel, McDonald's and the rest of Sydney's cheeky food offerings. Not until I got home did I realise that I did not even notice these places nor have the craving to eat at any of them. And believe me…the Krispy Kremes and McDonald's of the world elicit the same gooey-greasy smell every single day of the year. Yet I did not even pay a wink of attention to them. Why? Because my mind has turned itself off to the possibility of consuming such crap food. For weeks I have battled to give up all the chemical-filled crap that I have consumed in the past and, while it took some time, I finally won the battle. I am no psychologist, but I tried to objectively look at where my thought process started…to where it has come to today in order to point out the difference below:

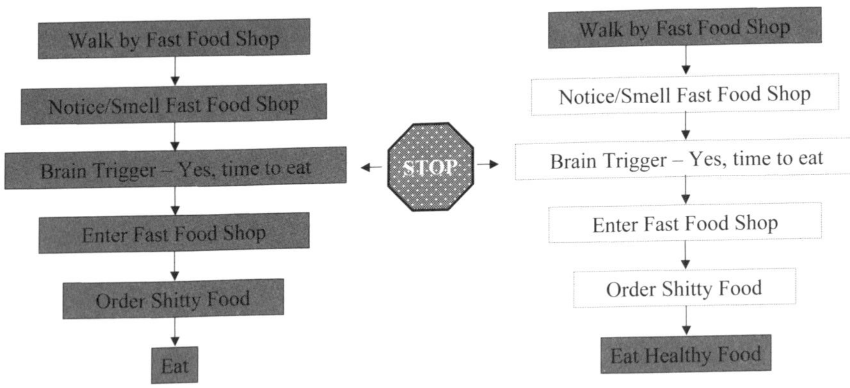

Figure A **Figure B**

Figure A is where I started pre-City Caveman Plan. 'Smell food, see food, eat food' was my diet plan. And as the boxes detail, I was the perfect fast food customer. I would carry on during my day, and first walk past a fast food shop as the greasy smell permeated through the air, my brain would trigger the natural response of 'Yes, time to eat!' So, I would walk in, place my order and indulge in my 60+ grams of fat.

Even during the early days of the City Caveman Plan, I had cravings for burgers, fries and fried chicken. I would still walk by the shops, notice and smell the food and my brain would trigger 'time to eat', yet due to my eating plan, I had to battle and suppress the urge to indulge, and say no to that brain trigger, which is why there is a stop sign. The first three steps were still there, but I just had to say no.

Today, that urge is completely gone, which is why Figure B has all the greyed-out boxes. I still walk by all the same shops, yet I do not even notice them or smell them. Therefore I have no urge to enter and order crap food. I have battled so many times this month, and won, that I have mentally and physically blocked out the urge to eat junk. How did I get there? Thirty-eight days of having a healthy eating plan and not deviating from it! In this plan, practice does not make perfect; practice makes damn good healthy habits.

It is a new feeling for me, but one I really enjoy.

Caveman Tip:

Battle, battle, battle…until you win. When you win the battle of food temptation, you move into a stage of control, which provides a new sense of balance.

Speaking of new feelings, my Bikram yoga day-after soreness is definitely noticeable. I am pretty sure I have stretched and strained some muscles that I have not used in the City Caveman Plan up to this point. And I am fine with that. It reminds me of when I do not play golf for quite a while: a day of eighteen holes means soreness the next day due to the use of muscles that are not normally strained and twisted on a daily basis. Bikram has hit my body in the same manner.

Thursday night is late night shopping in Sydney and, with the end-of-year sales, just about everything is reduced. My shopping style has normally been typical of a guy – I know what I need, I go to get what I need, buy it and go home. There is no perusing or browsing, no chatting with the sales folks, or catching up for coffee with mates in between purchases. I am a focused and determined shopper, and there is no need to waste time on any other distracting tasks.

That was, until now. With a new Caveman body, it has been so fantastic to rummage through all the sale clothes. I have moved from being a size XL to a Medium, and maybe I am a little biased, but it seems like everything looks good on me. I WANT TO BUY IT ALL!

It is a cool feeling to try on the tighter fitting t-shirts and ditching the styles I used to wear that hid my fat and looked like I was wearing a tent. I can now tuck in my shirts, and I can wear slimmer-fitting jeans – it's amazing. And though I really do not have the surplus dollars to be shopping, I don't care. A new body means I fully deserve some new clothes because I have earned it. My chubby-guy jeans are like an old skin to me, and it feels so good to shed them.

Day 40: my final day. Tomorrow. Wow.

Annie says: *Congratulations to Mike on winning the food battle as it is half the battle of the bulge. One half is fighting the junk food cravings, and the other half is fighting the urge for inactivity. Once you master those two battles, you have won the war against fat.*

I, too, enjoy a treat like a doughnut or a pizza every now and again, but I don't feel compelled to go into McDonalds and order a burger every time I walk past an outlet. Because, as Mike has come to realise, once you have been consistently eating healthy and feeling the positive effects of a clean diet, you become motivated to keep those positive effects rather than eating crap and feeling like you've undone all your hard work.

The other day I indulged in nachos for lunch, which was great until I got to the gym and started my run. My stomach was so clogged with corn chips and cheese that I felt too uncomfortable to keep going. Now that really annoyed me, so I won't be doing that again! Healthy food is digested faster and is rich in nutrients, so you are left with more energy to complete your workouts.

Splurging on some new clothes is a fantastic feeling, isn't it? Anybody who has gone through the City Caveman Plan and has been rewarded with a fabulous, new, sexy body deserves to look and feel as good as they can afford! The reward and congratulations for taking on a 40-day challenge is a new body and new clothes, which equates to an entirely new look.

Your friends, partner and family will all be pleasantly surprised, so consider their reactions a Caveman trophy.

Day 40. Not the Finish Line

> *I just want to see how long I can keep this thing going. The easiest thing is dying. Living is a pain in the butt.*
>
> – Jack LaLanne

There is torrential rain outside, but in my world there was nothing but sunshine!

Day 40 had arrived, and I could not believe I made it! Actually, I take that back because I worked damn hard to strictly follow the City Caveman Plan and win (almost) every battle I was faced with. It's a great feeling to be here!

Annie and I were going to do the Stairway to Hell today, but the clouds and rain would not allow for a final run, so off to the gym it was for me.

There was a hint of celebration in the air, so the workout was a very easy one.

Sonja and I later cooked up a celebratory meal of grilled salmon with garlic, soy, veggies and salad, followed by a nice bottle of wine on the town. We met some friends, had some laughs and a chat and enjoyed a great night out.

Of course, being at Day 40, my friends all asked whether I would return to my old ways.

Well, I guess that remains to be seen with time, but for now my answer is 'Hell no!' I did not take on this challenge to spend forty days just to prove to myself, my mates and Annie that I could take a short break from a life of destruction. I took it on as a way to negate my indulgent lifestyle, to learn about efficient workouts and to educate myself about clean consumption of fluids and food so I could apply it to my lifestyle permanently. It was not like I was on Survivor, where I lived in extreme conditions for a period in time, only to be returned at the end to my former life. For me, the City Caveman Plan was a 40-day learning period, designed to get my life back on the healthy track, for the long term.

Even though from Day 1 I was viewing today as the finish line, I realise now that it is anything but the finish line. In fact, it really is only the beginning; the beginning of my new, improved life.

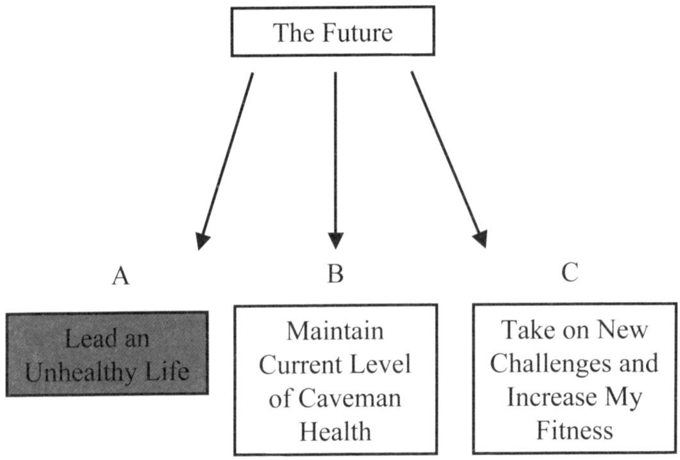

The City Caveman Plan has given me options that were not available to me prior to my improved health. As the chart above shows, the future can now go in one of three places for me: lead an unhealthy life, maintain my current level of caveman health, or I can take on new challenges and increase my fitness.

Lead an Unhealthy Life

Is this an option? Sadly, yes. I could trip up and hit the bars and bad food path again. It was my lifestyle before, so I could, potentially, fall back into it. However, I believe the forty days have given me the tools as well as the confidence to say goodbye to bad eating and dietary habits. This lifestyle is gone.

Maintain Current Level of Caveman Health

Yes, I could stay on the path I have lived for the past forty days. I would probably mix in a few more drinks and a couple of brie-and-biscuit evenings if I did, but I would be happy to maintain my current weight, fitness and mental state. I have conquered, and I have won, and so to maintain this feeling of mental and physical satisfaction would be a pretty good place to reside.

Take on New Challenges and Increase My Fitness

I feel that I am in the position to do whatever I want. Meaning, if I want to chase those six-pack abs, I can. If I want to enter a (mini) triathlon event, I could. I know

now that I have the abilities to take on those new battles, and win them. I am ready for the next level of health and fitness.

The City Caveman Plan took me off option A and revealed that there was a road to options B and C if I was willing to do the hard yards to get to them. And, after just forty days I now feel like I can do anything I want and win!

The future is here, and now I know I will continue to make the smartest choice to ensure I live a healthier life for the long-term.

Caveman Tip:

Look yourself in the mirror and decide today that health and fitness was not temporary but rather part of the new you. The *choice* is now yours.

Sonja and I had a great few glasses of wine at a swanky little wine bar with a couple of friends. It was a quiet, yet fantastic, celebration. And that is how my life is meant to be. I need to think of my drinking as a treat, rather than a social necessity. We shared a bottle, had a nice little buzz and came back for a Caveman cuddle.

Will I miss the City Caveman Plan? Yes and no. On one hand it is almost like saying goodbye to a friend who has taught me a lot. There have been ups and downs and battles, but also many victories. I have gone from fat to fit, so I love the City Caveman Plan and so, in that regard, yes, I will miss it. But, on the other hand it has been very challenging, and I took Sonja along for an often bumpy ride, so from that aspect, I am eager to say goodbye to the City Caveman Plan.

I feel like a university student at graduation. I am ready for the next chapter. I am a better person for every day I spent with the City Caveman Plan and, while forty days was the perfect amount of time to make a change, I am so excited for the next phase and challenge in my life.

Annie's Note to Mike:

Looking at you on Day 40, Fit Mike, I am so impressed and proud. Impressed, because you had the willpower and drive to complete the forty days, in the middle of winter when all your friends were doing the opposite, and you had little chance to show off your new body. And proud because I feel like I had a hand in moulding you into the man you are today: tanned, fit and fantastic. It is like a male version of 'My Fair Lady' only it's 'My Fair Caveman'. You must have a great sense of accomplishment.

Each day you ticked the boxes and got it done: the eating plan, the workouts and the water intake. And you did it without much complaining and no excuses. Job very well done. If you apply the same drive, commitment and enthusiasm to any new goal in the future, you are bound to be successful, because that is what success is: having a vision of what you want, creating a plan to achieve it and reaching the end of the rainbow and your goals, all while enjoying that journey.

And what impresses me most is not the new waistline or the new abs, but it is that you realise that this is not the conclusion but, rather, the beginning of a new life. It took forty days of living like a City Caveman, but you really do actually get it.

I hope you enjoy your pot of gold, because you truly deserve it, Mike. You deserve to live a healthy and fit life, you deserve the compliments and attention you've earned, and you deserve that celebratory glass of wine I know you'll enjoy.

I feel privileged to have taken this journey with you, and for your results I give you my admiration and respect.

I am going to have a glass of wine myself, to salute us and the next forty days and beyond. May we live them all as happily and healthily as we have in the last forty!

15

But Wait, There's More!

Do not put this book down yet – because we are not quite done! Remember, Yogi Berra said: It's not over 'til it's over.

If you have read to this page, then you've probably just finished your own 40-day journey, so CONGRATULATIONS! You made it!

Forty days of Caveman change, forty days of battling and forty days of no drinking. So, I hope you, like me, have celebrated with a glass of wine (or two) and toasted our great accomplishment of committing, performing and achieving!

So, why aren't we done then? Because, although the City Caveman Plan is successfully completed, we still have to chat about the next phase: the Control Phase.

By taking on the City Caveman Plan we learned how to say 'goodbye' to the Abuse Phase. We then spent a good forty days battling and succeeding within the Change Phase, and now that our forty days are completed, we have successfully graduated to the Control Phase. And it is here that we should start to think about what could tempt us to fall back into the Abuse Phase.

It can take years to construct a building, what with the planning, the materials and the construction process; yet it only takes a few days to blow it up in a spectacular fashion. Our bodies are similar. We've put in so much work and won so many battles in the past forty days, but it only takes a few weeks of explosive eating and drinking to fall right back into the Abusive Phase and start that Obesity Snowball rolling again.

So, let's give some thought on how to enter into and succeed in the Control Phase, so we can enjoy our health and our new lives for the long term.

The Control Phase

I know; you may have thought the Caveman battles had ended, but a new battle has begun. The new battle is all about *control*.

Control is not just about the forty days we've just lived through; it's actually more about the next forty days, the forty days after those and the next forty days after those.

We have successfully managed to alter our behaviour to reach our goal of living in the Change Phase for forty days, so the next challenge is to work out how to maintain similar Caveman control for rest of our lives! Think about this:

- Are you feeling stronger?
- Are you leaner?
- Are you healthier?
- Is your skin better?
- Are you more confident about your body?
- Are you happier?

If, like me, the answer is 'yes', then don't you *want* to continue to control your behaviour so you can keep feeling this great? I know I do!

We Have Changed...So That We Can Control

The City Caveman Plan is not like implementing a new accounting system over a 40-day period, because the City Caveman Plan has no end. Yes, we have ended our time in the Change Phase, but the Control Phase is actually even more important. Why? Because although it is the last phase in this program, it is also a never-ending battle. In order to retain this healthy life, we need to control our intake of food, make sure we have hangover-free days and continue to have effective workouts for the rest of our lives.

I never wanted to tell my story so that it sounded like I had 'graduated' from the City Caveman Plan just because I managed to jump over a 40-day hurdle. Instead, the point was always to create a timed phase that would allow myself to change my lifestyle, learn about a new and healthier lifestyle, and then, afterwards, understand how to make this lifestyle permanent. Because now, on Day 40+, I have the choice to control my lifestyle, enjoy my health and continue living in this healthy zone forever – if I want to.

Having spent so many years tearing my body down, now that I have rebuilt it with healthy foundations I refuse to return to that Abusive Phase. My Obesity Snowball has stopped, and I am going to live a healthy life for many years to come. Of course, I am still going to eat pizza and drink alcohol occasionally, but the battle now becomes: how do I reintroduce the cheeky things into my life without restarting the rolling of my Obesity Snowball? It's up to me to choose my path.

Here are some Australian statistics to put it into perspective:[viii]

- Sixty per cent of our population is overweight.
- Every year our public hospitals treat 500,000 people for preventable illnesses.
- Every year over 50,000 people die from illnesses caused by their poor lifestyle.
- A National Heart Foundation study estimates that seven lifestyle factors – obesity, low fruit and vegetable consumption, tobacco use, alcohol consumption, low physical activity, high cholesterol and high blood pressure – cause 52,738 deaths in Australia every year, accounting for 39 per cent of all deaths.
- One in six Australians (3.5 million of us) suffers from cardiovascular disease. It's costing our health system $7.6 billion a year and by 2050 it is estimated that one in four will be affected.
- More than one million Australians currently have the lifestyle-related type-2 diabetes. By 2030 that number will more than double. And one of the main factors contributing to all this ill health is our weight.

---

viii Dunlevy, Sue, 2007, 'Fat Chance of Living a Healthy Life', <http://blogs.news.com.au/dailytelegraph/suedunlevy/index.php/dailytelegraph/comments/fat_chance_of_living_healthy_life/>.

- Experts estimate that obesity is responsible for 102,000 cases of diabetes, 379,000 cases of cardiovascular disease, 20,000 cases of cancer and 225,000 cases of osteoarthritis every year.

Think about it. When it comes to our health, 60 per cent of us are facing potential heart problems, diabetes and other possibly life-threatening illnesses if we do not make the right health choices.

Which path do you want to go down?

The Caveman Choice

Forty days ago we were unhealthy, eating poorly and not working out. We really didn't allow ourselves a choice of health because we were so deeply embedded in living a life of bad habits. Our Obesity Snowball was gaining momentum and we had nothing in place to stop it.

Yet after forty days? Well, we've kicked those bad habits, learned and adopted new good habits, become active, increased our fitness – we've given ourselves a new life and we've now rewarded ourselves with opportunities to do whatever we want. For many of us, *choices* have become the biggest rewards from the City Caveman Plan.

With our new body and a new mindset, we now have the choice to take our lives in any direction we want; if we want to enter a 10km race, start bike riding or hiking, we can now do all of those things. The key choice is, of course, to never return to our obese lifestyle and choose to travel with the healthier, happier 40 per cent.

I spoke about it in Day 40 as well: I love the empowering result of the City Caveman Plan as we have now given ourselves this choice. Sure, we can choose to go back to our old lifestyle, but we have given ourselves the tools to avoid that road and even continue on to a healthier lifestyle. We taught ourselves to read food labels, to listen to our body during workouts and, most of all, we showed the dedication to change. And now that we have changed, it is up to us to control – this is the next battle, and it is one I am going to win because I found my own Happy-Healthy Zone, the zone where I choose to live.

The Happy-Healthy Zone

What is the Happy-Healthy Zone? It's that zone where I now respect my body, cherish my health and make the right choices in order to maintain both of these. It's not about perfection, nor is it about 'the look' that's hot in social circles. It's that zone where I can look myself in the mirror and feel the mind/body confidence that I feel in leading a healthy, positive life. There are other health zones in which people can choose to live, as the chart details below, but the Happy-Healthy Zone is ideally where all of us should aim to be.

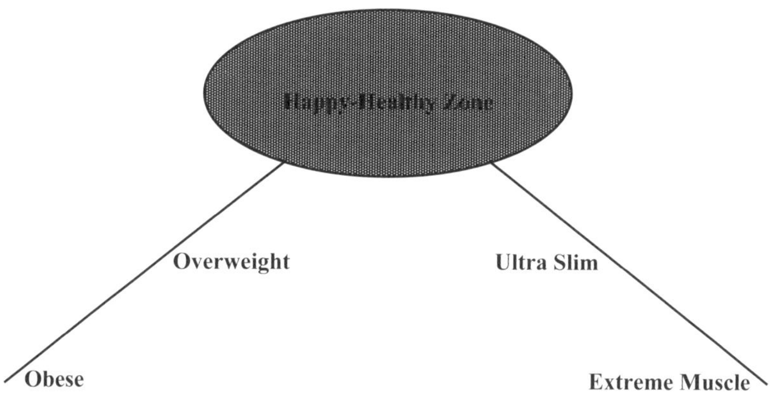

The Ultra Slim and Extreme Muscle Group

I believe that those who strive to be ultra slim or super muscular are living in the extremes, which is damn hard work. These people are often chasing their perceived image of perfection, but to that I say, 'Bullshit!' I'm *not* chasing perfection, but instead merely want to look good in a t-shirt and a pair of jeans. It is this level of mind/body confidence that I strive for.

The Obese and Overweight Group

This is where I started (along with 60 per cent of us in Australia!). I know this group too well; we don't watch what we eat, we are not getting enough exercise. I don't want to ever be a part of this group again.

The Happy-Healthy Zone

I'm happy, I'm healthy and I'm in a zone I don't want to leave. Perfect? Well, no, but I'm perfectly happy by *my* standards, not those in a magazine or in a movie. Perfection is not about being visually sculpted or about obtaining a number on my biceps; to me, it's about my state of health and the way I feel towards myself. And my zone will differ from Bob or Jane's Happy-Healthy Zone. It's the individual pleasure in knowing we have our health and our lives under control.

There's a reason the chart on the prior page is circular in shape, and that's because the Happy-Healthy Zone is not about an ideal weight, or an ideal state of mind, or about obtaining a certain look. It's about finding our own state of mind and body happiness while living a healthy lifestyle; our own mental comfort zone in knowing that we're leading an overall healthy life.

If I'm living in my Happy-Healthy Zone, then a one-kilogram weight gain here or there shouldn't stress me out because I am not chasing perfection or the next blockbuster movie role. I just want to maintain my mind and body confidence, and so, unlike the person chasing that extreme image, one kilogram is not going to shake that for me because I now have access to plenty of healthy recipes and good workouts when and if I want to lose that kilogram.

The idea behind the Control Phase is to always live in that Happy-Healthy Zone where you can enjoy life without sacrificing your health in the process – to moderately enjoy the Sunday barbecues with a sausage and a couple of beers, a few slices of pizza, but also to enjoy a nice 5km run in the sun or a long beach walk close to the ocean. It's about taking pride in your appearance and health and to continue to perform the physical measures necessary to stay comfortable and smiling within that Happy-Healthy Zone.

Of course, it's also about understanding behaviour that might pose a threat to falling out of that zone so, in a bid to help minimise these risks, I have created some steps to ensure that I never start that Obesity Snowball rolling ever again.

16

Maintaining the Happy-Healthy Zone

By putting these six ideas into action, we can all stay happy and healthy for the long term:

Develop a Caveman Conscience

While at the supermarket tonight, I was in the mood for a cheeky snack, so I made my way down the chip aisle, where I noticed the corn chips and dip, the different potato chip options and all those little orange cheesy ball things. Call it habit or conditioning from forty days in the Change Phase, but I walked past the cheesy snack with its 25 grams of fat and, instead, opted for some whole-wheat, baked pretzels, saving myself about 20 grams of fat in the process. I subconsciously battled, and I made the right choice.

After making the pretzel purchase, I realised that I had developed a Caveman Conscience.

Pre-City Caveman Plan, I would see chips, buy chips and eat chips (most often before I even got to the checkout and paid for them!). But, with my new Caveman Conscience, I can now see those chips, but instead of immediately tearing them open and shovelling them into my mouth, I think about my health and search for a healthier option that will still satisfy my hunger or tastebud's desires.

It is decisions like that that my heart, my skin and my weight will all thank me for in the long run, and that is what the Caveman Conscience is about; the extra consideration and patience when thinking about food choices. It's about seeing the unhealthy Eggs Benedict but smartly choosing the poached eggs on toast. It's about ignoring the fat-laden Caesar salad dressing and selecting one of the tasty, low-fat Caveman Recipe options.

Whatever meal I am shopping for, I need to recruit my Caveman Conscience to help me see what's good, fresh and healthy in order to keep making the right choices to retain my healthy life and leaner body.

Stay Active and Make it a Lifestyle

The City Caveman Plan was not a trial period for exercise. It was about making a plan, sticking to that exercise plan and realising that cardio work and resistance training is exactly what I needed to lower my weight and regain my health.

So why would I stop my workouts now?

I won't. I won't because I like it, because I enjoy it and because I need exercise in my life to keep this body in its new shape and to retain this new level of health and fitness.

Life is so much better with this improved body, and exercise has now become an enjoyable part of my lifestyle, so I don't want to let it go.

I like the way I look now. I like my new body, and I like knowing that I can enjoy a cheeky meal because it will be worked off at the gym on the following day. I understand that I can only maintain this balance and, therefore, my Happy-Healthy Zone, if I keep my body moving and stay active – so that's what I will do.

Remember the Journey

The best thing about a rags-to-riches story is when the individual who makes good remains humble and is able to take what he's learned from his journey and apply it to the rest of his life. And while the City Caveman Plan is not quite a rags-to-riches story, in a similar fashion I don't ever want to forget my fat-to-fit journey either.

Whether it's my workouts, my eating, or my drinking, I have developed new patterns and a new lifestyle, so it's important to remember where I started and to remind myself of the challenging process of change, so that I never trip up and find myself back at Day 1 of the City Caveman Plan.

Workouts

I started my City Caveman Plan with low-energy, hangover-inspired workouts. Yet the City Caveman Plan has turned my workouts around completely, so that nowadays I give 100 per cent effort, after having fuelled my body properly, and I enter the gym with the Game Day mindset. Add to that a plan that Annie and I created, and BAM – fantastic workouts and awesome results!

Eating

My eating patterns of the past were nothing short of terrible. But, in forty days, I've transformed my lifestyle where I'm enjoying nutritious meals that are full of flavour, and that are also giving me the energy I need to perform at the level I want during my workouts.

These days I almost feel like an explorer, seeking new recipes, researching healthy ways to create delicious meals and getting a feel for what my body likes and positively responds to. This 'newness' is both fun and exciting, and I have found myself taking pride, not only in the way I look but also in the fact I now have a full fruit and veggie bowl at home, as well as a refrigerator full of fresh, non-processed, tasty food. I don't want this feeling to end.

Drinking

My biggest transformation, which will continue to be my biggest ongoing battle, is in my drinking habits.

As you know, drinking itself isn't the only challenge for me; additionally, it's the drinking that turns into the late-night kebab, which turns into bad sleep, which turns into a bad hangover, which turns into poor exercise. So for me, the key to a successful post-City Caveman Plan is to restrict my drinking to celebratory drinks only.

So what are celebratory drinks?

Celebratory drinks are those 'after-work' drinks after a hard working week, or when you drink to celebrate a mate's birthday party, or while you watch a DVD over a bottle of wine with a loved one. It will never again be about the huge midweek night out, the solo bottle of wine for no real reason, or the pub-crawls that conclude with a double burger and large fries. It will be difficult, it will be a battle, but I now think am at least armed with the ability to make the right choice.

The food battles, temptations and cravings were difficult, but the change shows in my new confidence and body. I am determined to remember the effort I put into this journey to make permanent the changes that I have made.

Choose My Deviance Wisely

In this Control Phase, I need to choose my deviance wisely by planning a healthy week. For example if I indulge in a poker, beer and pizza night with the boys on Friday, then I need to have a healthy and drink-free Monday, Tuesday, Wednesday and Thursday. Similarly, if there's a farewell celebration on Sunday afternoon for a mate who's travelling overseas, then I need to have a DVD Saturday night in, with a fresh salmon dinner and a Sunday morning beach run. In essence, it's the way to have my cake and eat it too! Yum! And to be honest, I think cheeky food or a few drinks will go down so much better when I know that those kilos won't stick to my side because I will be too busy running them off the very next day, or I will have prepared myself wisely by earning it the day before. By learning how to schedule in advance, and plan a bit better, and by not being afraid to say 'no' to some social events, my health will benefit.

In order to win this battle I need to make a conscious effort to strengthen my weakness, and I know that this will take time and continued hard work. But, I remember hearing a golf announcer talk about Tiger Woods once and he said something along the lines of, 'Tiger's strength is in his weakness. He figures out his own weaknesses and then practises and tweaks those weaknesses until they become part of his artillery of strengths.'

If I follow that strategy to keep practising until my former weaknesses become second-nature strengths, then I should soon have no troubles choosing deviances that will keep me within my Happy-Healthy Zone.

Stay Accountable

I love the Caveman Contract that I signed as well as the daily tick box chart that was on my mirror. If it wasn't the verbal tongue-lashing I would have received from Annie had I quit during my forty days, it was the disappointment I would have felt looking myself in the mirror knowing I could not tick the boxes in my City Caveman Plan that would have left me feeling down and depressed. I felt like the accountability measures were essential and extremely effective to ensure I did not fall off track.

Sure, at times, I felt like a bit of a goof to have this tick box piece of paper on my bathroom mirror, but it did help me take on a new mentality that will stay with me in the years to come; it taught me about taking full responsibility and becoming the CEO of both my health and my body.

A CEO presides over hundreds, sometimes thousands, of people. That CEO controls his or her business and continually makes decisions to determine the health of the corporation. And if the shit hits the fan? It's that CEO who is on the news taking the blame. And when high profits are announced? That same CEO reaps the monetary rewards for the good decisions made. Whether good or bad, the CEO has the responsibility for the company that he or she governs and takes full accountability for its actions.

Like a company, I will battle to become the CEO of my own body. Just as a corporate CEO needs to control his company, I need to think about controlling my body and what goes into it in order to achieve the results I want in the end. By battling and becoming the CEO of my body, I will be able to govern it wisely and hold myself accountable, stay fit and enjoy my new, healthy lifestyle.

Because...Because I Have To

When I was a child, I would typically ask the teacher something like 'Why do I have to do this science homework? I hate science.' To which, my teacher would usually reply, 'You will study science, Michael, because you have to.'

In trying to stay in my Happy-Healthy Zone, if I forget to stay accountable or forget my fat-to-fit journey, or if I forget all the other steps I've already mentioned, then I will simply revert to my school teacher's simplistic logic in order to keep myself in the Happy-Healthy Zone, by remembering those wise words:

I must stay healthy...because I have to.

Because it's the best way to live.
Because it's a good example for our children.
Because having material things means nothing if I don't have my health.
Because it's no fun being ill.
Because I owe it to my family to be around for a while.
Because improving quality of life is fucking important.
Because the cost of healthcare is out of control.
Because it makes life more fun.
Because I look younger, fresher and better.
Because taking medication sucks.
Because I was born healthy, and that is an amazing gift that I should honour.

Simply, because I have to.

17

Day 45 – The Before and The After

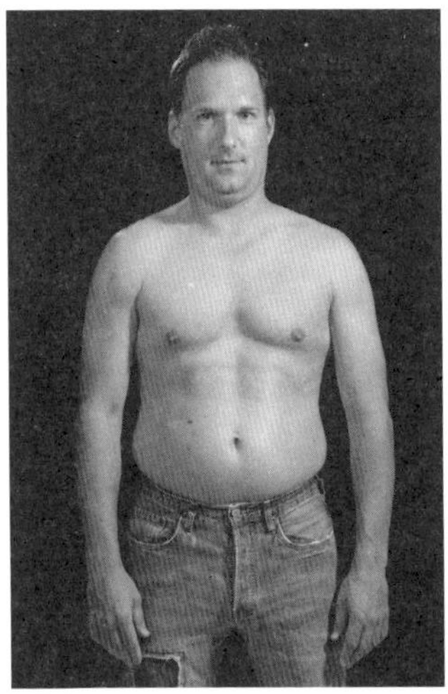

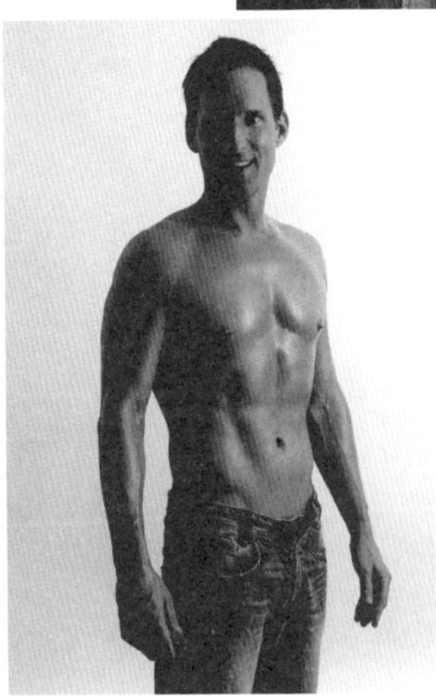

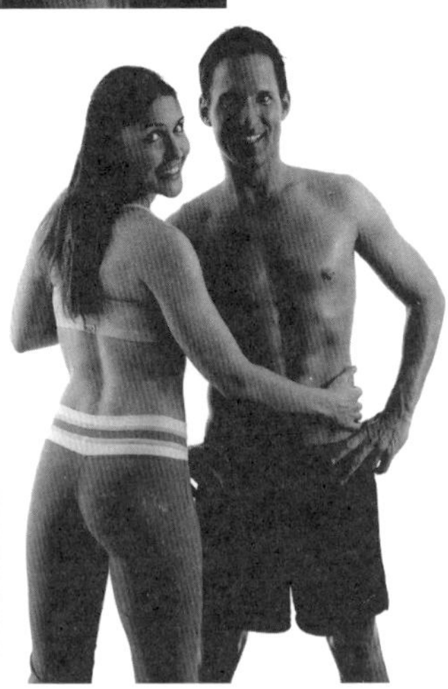

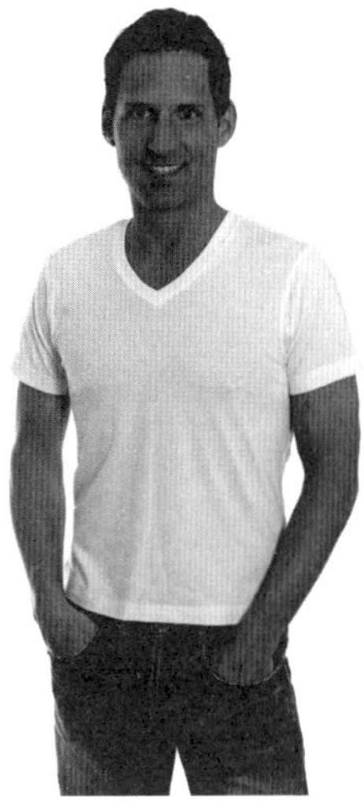

The Photos

Annie says: *What else can I say, but 'WOW'! What a turnaround!*

If a picture tells a thousand words, then I think Mike's could be closer to the million-word range. I am very, very proud of his dedication and accomplishment as he looks great and he feels even better. These photos and his new body are his reward for staying true to the City Caveman Plan.

A few years back, I was featured in a monthly fitness magazine, whereby one body part at a time was featured over a 12-month period, and I wrote about the exercises needed for readers to obtain 'Annie's legs' and so on. It was quite a flattering feature, so in a similar spirit I thought it would be good to detail and describe Mike's 'After' body in the same fashion.

The Mental – Change

My initial thought was to work through Mike's photos and start remarking about specific parts of his newly improved body – the abs, the arms, the shoulders, etc. However, I don't only see the BODY; more than anything I witnessed the emotional and mental changes that Mike went through, and this change cannot really be identified in a photo showcasing new muscles or poses.

Mike battled and won. I did not receive endless calls from him whingeing that it was too difficult a challenge, as he was truly motivated to make a change from Day 1 on. And in fitness, the mind is like a waterfall: once it changes, the rest flows downward and the body is able to change accordingly, so I kept telling Mike to envision himself as the fit guy on the cover of a men's health magazine. I kept telling him to say 'I am fit, I am fit' over and over again as he was conquering his daily Mount Everest-type challenges. These positive thoughts gave him direction and gave him a goal – he did not just go through the daily motions of a workout, but, instead, he mentally transformed himself into something he wanted to become.

But, in saying this, it was not an overnight transformation. I remember trying to calm Mike down on the phone, after the self-photography session following Week 1, and believe me – he was one furious Caveman. When making such drastic life changes, it is not uncommon for individuals to feel disappointed when results are not immediately seen, but this was just another of the many battles that Mike overcame triumphantly. And while he may have felt discouraged at that point in time, I was on the other end of the phone, quietly and positively encouraged. Why? Because while he was focused on the mirror, I was focused on the encouraging aspects of his first week:

- *Mike changed all his eating patterns in a one-week period,*
- *he changed his drinking patterns in that one-week period,*
- *he completed and battled through a week of tough workouts, and*
- *most importantly, Mike was motivated to continue on into Week 2.*

Roll these four factors into Week 2 and Week 3 and you are looking at a time period where bad habits turn into good habits – where mentally, you have progressed and slightly transformed. Then, continue these factors into Week 4, Week 5 and Week 6, and it's a certainty that physical and mental changes would start to embed themselves.

Fitness and change do not occur with the blink of an eye; it is all a process and, at times, a gruelling and frustrating one. For some, that process is longer than others, but the challenge to change one's lifestyle is the same for all. And the beauty of this mind/body change lies further away than the photos because, subconsciously, Mike now knows that if he puts his mind toward a project or a goal, he has the confidence that he will accomplish it.

And this is because his life, not just his body, has changed as a direct result of the City Caveman Plan.

The Physical – Face

I am a firm believer that health can be seen in the eyes, and Mike's eyes now show life to me. Backing up forty days ago when we were discussing where Mike was at the present, he would talk about his own health and fitness and tend to look downward while conversing with me. This was a definite sign that Mike lacked confidence in himself. I could also look into his eyes, back then, and see how unhealthy his body was; the hangovers, the bad sleep and the bad food were all visible in his eyes.

However, that has all changed now. Mike now has whiter, healthier looking eyes that reflect the past forty healthy days of no alcohol, no hangovers and great workouts.

While men usually pay no attention to the health and texture of their skin, Mike's looks fantastic. This is because of the detoxification that occurred over the 40-day period. Erasing the fried food, alcohol and the soft drinks that are filled with chemicals and replacing them with healthy veggies, fresh fruit and lean meats has detoxed his entire body and allowed him to battle that anti-ageing monster head on, leaving him with glowing, healthy, flawless skin; another battle (and one he may not even have known he was fighting) won!

Moving on to, well, the obvious, actually: Mike's double chin. No more gobble-gobble-gobble! Okay, I don't mean to be harsh on Mike, but as I am laying down all of these compliments, I can now give him a hard time about the 'before' photo. Seriously – what a change. The round, chubby cheeks with a second chin has turned into a slim/lean face with a distinct jaw line. The transition from his head to his neck/body is aesthetically more attractive. He started out with that 'thick head, thick neck, thick body' look of a guy who hits the pubs way too often, and now he has the well-defined face and wears the look of a fit and lean gym goer.

The eyes, the jaw line, the skin – Mike has given himself a new face that shows health, change and happiness.

The Physical – Arms and Shoulders

Even without taking scientific measurements, I can see the body fat decreases in Mike's shoulders and arms. Forty days prior, his arms just kind of hung and flailed off a chubby frame. Now, his arms are firm and they are noticeable. I know Mike said he did not want to turn into Arnold Schwarzenegger but, like most guys, he hoped to get bigger arms and expressed this a few times over the forty days. Did his arms get bigger? Can he curl more weight? Yes. But our eating and fitness plan was not designed to put on muscles on top of muscles.

Body builders consume specific muscle-building diets in order to build their arms, which takes time. Forty days to pump up your arms? I told Mike that this would not occur in our City Caveman Plan. But in saying that, his arms and shoulders are noticeably bigger, definitely stronger, and they suit his lean/fit body perfectly. He is now at the stage where he obtained that lean and slim frame. And if he wants to build big arms? He can do it, although, as they are, those arms and shoulders already look healthy, fit and fantastic.

The Physical – Chest and Abs

Okay, I have managed to refrain from swearing too much during my writing, but when I look at these photos, I have to say: Holy Shit!

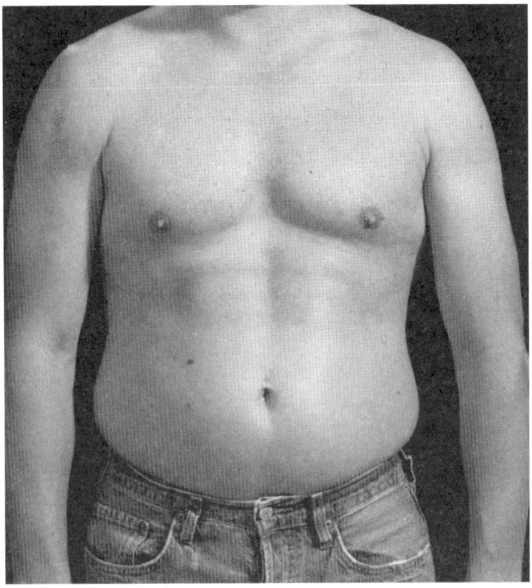
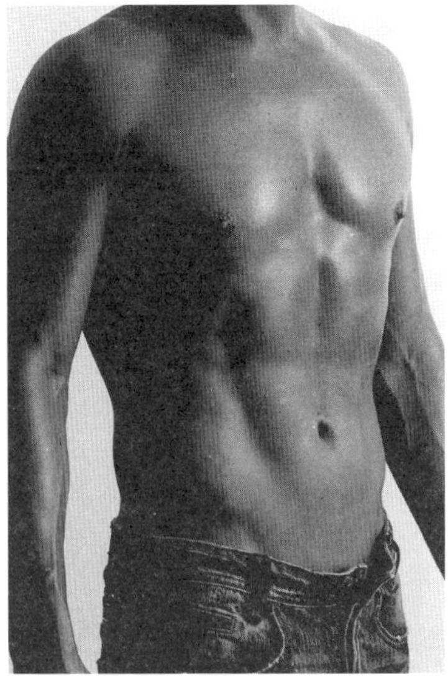

Physically, I can see change-change-change-change-change in every centimetre of these photos. The before/after difference? Well, do I really need to state the obvious?

You can see that Mike went from a pear-shape to V-shape, with his man boobs transforming into a defined chest, and his barrel-pack changing into a six-pack stomach. And while they say it's what is inside that matters, in that 'before' photo, what is inside is too many chemicals, bad circulation and overall poor health. But now? Mike is filled only with healthy nutrients, water and lean muscle. The 'before' photo is the work of time in the pub and late-night takeaway, while the 'after' photos are the results of hard work in the gym and healthy home-cooked meals.

Can you see that even Mike's posture has changed? The slouching posture that he developed when he was unhealthy and unfit is gone now, being replaced with a more upright and confident stance. Some of it is physical, as his chest/back muscles have re-shaped his entire upper half, and some of it is mental as well: his mind/body change has made him more confident so he, naturally, tends to stand taller.

If anybody ever wants to know the answer to these questions…

- *What will reducing your alcohol consumption do?*
- *What will good cardio workouts do for you?*
- *What does a lower fat diet do for you?*
- *What will I look like after performing an efficient, full body exercise regime?*

…the answer is in Mike's 'after' photos. To increase the look of your core muscles, you must watch your diet, drink less alcohol and fizzy drinks, and workout your body; it is that simple.

Switching gears a little, the societal issue that really irks me personally is television. Shows that glorify cosmetic surgery might have taken a look at Mike forty days ago and immediately said: Let's get a bit of liposuction here, there and a bit over here as well and we'll get you that V-shape back in no time at all.

Well, to hell with that plan and to the 'easy fix' that proclaims to do the same thing in such an easy way. Why does it irk me so much? Because look at the change he made in forty days. It's only forty days! He did not undergo anaesthesia, and he did not sign up for risky surgery. Mike simply made a change in his lifestyle and did it the gratifying way. Most importantly, the result of this path is that he learned what it takes to get it done. Undergoing surgery to reduce your beer gut only teaches you that money buys a new body. But if all you did was sign the bottom of the cheque to get that new body, well, I would put big dollars on it that that beer belly will be back in no time at all. You can't have the physical, unless you make the change mentally, and this is where surgery goes amiss.

The Future

Mike knows what it takes to physically change his body, but more importantly, he now appreciates what changes are required mentally to achieve such a large goal.

It may sound odd, but 'change' is now his, and he can take it wherever he wants. In the forty days he has gone from the initial chubby chap to a lean, fit City Caveman.

One never knows what their transformation will look like in the end, but now that Mike has achieved this goal for himself, it is truly up to him what he wants to do with it.

If he wants to turn into a runner, or if he wants to gain more muscle mass then it can all be achieved. The City Caveman Plan has given him the options to go anywhere he wants to go. He is comfortable in his Happy-Healthy Zone, and I know he will stay that way wherever his next challenge leads him because it makes him feel so good to be there.

18

The Photography Battle – Becoming Hairless

I had given up alcohol, pizza, cheese and so much more over a 40-day period, and now it was time to give up my hair. Ugh.

First off, Annie suggested I head to the tanning booth for a couple of sessions to improve upon my ghost-like tan prior to the photos. This one, I could handle; after all, she is the one that has done fitness modelling, so all I could do was take her advice on how to look my best for my photos. And after seeing my milky white skin in the first photo, I secretly thought she was right to suggest I take the edge off my Casper the Friendly Ghost pigmentation.

Somehow though, the conversation then took a turn, to sound something like this:

> 'Hey, what else should I do to get ready for the photos tomorrow?'
> 'Go hairless.'
> 'Pardon me?'
> 'Shave, wax, whatever, but just take off all your hair so we can see you fully exposed.'
> 'Ummmmm, are you serious? All, um, over my body?'
> 'Yes Mike. All over.'
> 'Shit. Okay.'

So, I went to the grocery store to find a host of hair removal products – wax strips, foams, sprays, gels; how in the hell would a guy know what to use? I just knew that ripping wax strips off my body was completely out of the question. In the end I bought some pink bottled hair-removing shaving cream-esque canister as well as a creamy roll-on contraption just to make sure I had enough. This was going to be a horrific chore.

I went home, dropped my gear and went to the bathroom. According to the directions, the shaving cream-esque canister was to be applied, then I had to wait five minutes and then wipe it off and watch the hair disappear. Sounds easy enough, right? Wrong.

After foaming up my legs, I settled in for that five-minute wait; standing naked in the middle of my bathroom I felt a little foolish. With nothing else to read I soon decided to suss out the side of the can to pass the time. The label read, 'Do not put foam on the nipple or reproductive area.' Before I could breathe a sigh of relief that I'd spared those areas, I started to feel a burning sensation in my testicles. They must have brushed up against my leg, transferring some of the foam onto *my boys*. I went into the shower to wipe it all off, only to find that when I went to do so, the hair on my legs wasn't falling out with ease like the box promised, but instead, remained fully attached but now in clump-like condition all the way up and down my legs!

The stinging sensation in my mid-section lasted for a few hours, which was about the same amount of time I took to shave my legs and body with a good old fashioned razorblade. What an ordeal!

This was definitely the first, and the last, time I would be going hairless! Though I did develop a new respect for women along the way!

The Photos

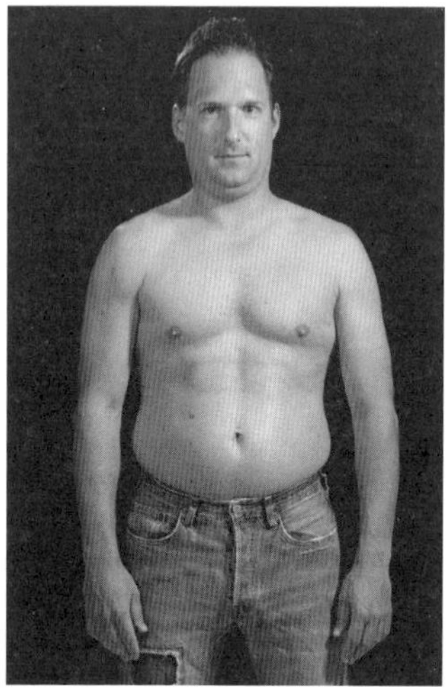

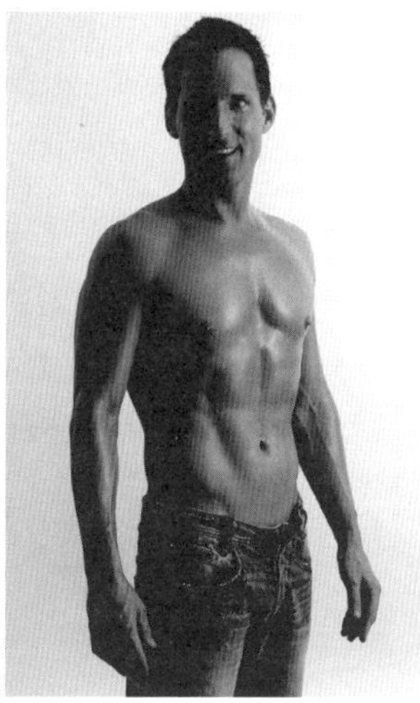

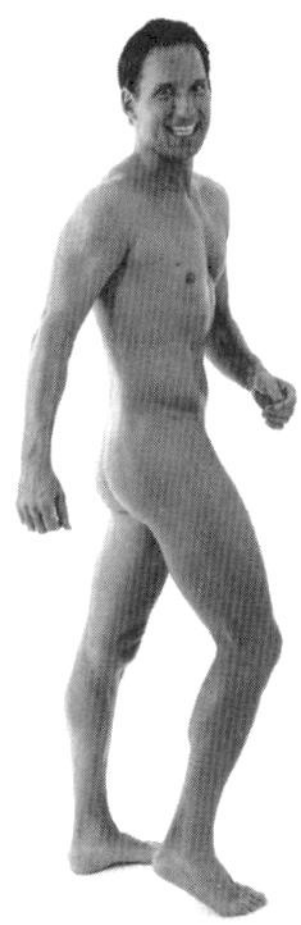

Well, like Annie said, 'Holy shit.'

Honestly. I really cannot believe my photos. And I don't mean that in a cocky way; I am truly humbled by what I see in those photos.

Is it really me in those pictures? It is such a strange sensation to see myself in these photos, but looking makes me determined to never let the chubby chap of the past return. Because I want to look like that guy in the 'after' photos - forever!

I think that although I feel great, and I know that I have psychologically changed a great deal, it really is the new body that astounds me the most at the moment. And that seems like the largest of all the changes that I've achieved.

Seeing these photos, I realise that the chubby chap in all of us hates being in photos; you can see the 'I'm so embarrassed, get me out of here' look in my face in that 'before' photo can't you? When we don't feel our best or look our best, we tend to avoid having our photo taken, because we do not want to have to look at what we truly are. I'll admit that even forty days ago, when I looked in the mirror I did not see the guy who's in the 'before' photo. Mainly because I didn't want to.

How I Feel

I feel fantastic, and I feel accomplished. I really did it, and the photos are my trophy.

I truly had no idea that I would be in this position, with this drastically new look. The change is amazing. And before anybody busts my balls and says 'Photoshop', I will retort before the words can be spoken, because except for digitally taking out a few freckles on my body and a couple of sessions in the tanning booth – what you see is entirely my body. It is me. I told our patient photographer that I wanted a true representation of my body, and he gave it to us in what you see before you.

Being naked was quite an experience, and while I am glad I did it (it was actually quite liberating to feel so comfortable being naked for once), you won't be seeing me in any nudie magazines any time in the near future! Unfortunately, my Mum back in the USA did not think the photo was so amazing. I think she prefers the bare skin, baby-on-the-rug type shots to be kept within the family! Oh well!

Thinking back, I remember Annie telling me throughout the month to envision myself as a guy on the cover of a fitness magazine, and that is what I would become. I kind of looked at her with a 'why are you telling me this psychological mumbo-jumbo?' because I really did not believe I could transform my thinking so radically. However, I think the photos show that I did manage to overcome my fears and, truth be known, I am ecstatic with the end results.

Before and After Statistics

Now, while I prefer to look at the differences in the photos and the changes in how I feel mentally and emotionally, these things cannot be measured statistically. So for those of you who really need numbers and digits as evidence of my achievement, here they are:

	40 Day Caveman Change		
	Day 1	**Day 40**	**Change**
Weight	88kgs	75kgs	15%
Body Fat	27.50%	13.00%	53%
Belly Button Circumference	44	32	27%
Jeans Size	36	31	14%
Cir-gut-ference Difference	1.22	1.03	16%

Stepping onto the scale on the morning of the photo shoot to see 75kgs was indescribable. To keep tap-tap-tapping the weight calibre to the left to get the appropriate weight was such an exciting feeling; it was so good to see the scales confirm that I had achieved what I set out to do.

My body fat fell from 27.5 per cent down to 13 per cent, which is apparently great, but all I really care most about is that photogenically and in my own head, I am no longer a fatty! The numbers merely confirm it on paper.

As for my Cir-gut-ference (which is a term I am proud to say I made up myself!), I was really happy to see this statistic improve so much. Mainly because I'd kind of told Annie that I would judge myself on the Cir-gut-ference ratio results, and also because deep down, even though we men may joke about our oversized guts (some of us even name them like they're our friend!), we most often despise it and wish it was gone every day of our lives. So I really did want to confirm that I had bid farewell to that long-term 'friend' of mine.

Some mates have asked me how they can get a six-pack too. I think people have the misconception that it takes crunches on top of crunches in order to obtain six-pack abs, but that is only partially correct. Certainly, it takes controlled, precise abdominal exercises in order to build muscle, but it also comes down to a low-fat diet to expose the muscles that you have under there. Because, if you have layers of fat on top of them then it doesn't matter how many muscles you create with crunches; the fat will always hide them! So, if a six-pack is what you want, remember that it is a combination of exercises to build the muscles, as well as a low-fat diet, that creates a *window* for them to be exposed.

Before the City Caveman Plan, when trying on clothes I'd head straight to the XL rack to ensure whatever I bought would hide my protruding gut. But after the Caveman Plan? I can now buy a tighter fitting Medium-sized shirt, which shows off my shoulders a bit more, yet still fits loosely down around my waist, highlighting that V-shaped body I now have!

I am swimsuit ready. I can take my shirt off while going for a run, and I can even feel confident in photos where I don't have my shirt on. Fit and healthy is definitely the way I want to stay.

Annie said it, the photos show it, the numbers confirm it and so now I can proudly say it too: I have changed.

19

My 35th Birthday

Yesterday was the 23rd of June, and it was my 35th birthday.

Please pardon my language, but I feel fucking fantastic.

Mentally and physically, I feel like I am a new person. I look great and I feel fit – it is as if somebody has turned the lights on in my life. I did not use any gimmicks, industry secrets or super athletic drugs to aid in my performance. I am most proud because in objectively looking at my lifestyle, I stripped out all the shit in my life, and I went back to the basics in order to make a 180 degree change in the direction of my health. I have made such a profound change in my life because of the simplicity with which I have chosen to live: healthy eating, no alcohol abuse and simple, yet effective, workouts.

But certainly, my journey was not easy.

In my daily workouts, I battled. I overcame my fear of weights, and I did not go through each day with a 'lose weight while doing this simple, easy exercise' infomercial smile. Instead I changed my mentality at the gym. Yet the battles became a bit easier as my mind and body progressed, and even the battles changed. Instead of weight room insecurities, just a few weeks later I was climbing my own Mount Everest; and I was winning.

In giving up bad food, I battled. Week 1 scents of fried food would send me into a frenzy. Giving up my order-the-tastiest-thing-on-the-menu-with-no-regard-to-health eating plan was not easy. Yet a 40-day plan of healthy, tasty eating changed my taste buds as well as my mental process in choosing my daily menu. And because of that, my whole outlook on what constitutes proper food consumption has changed.

In giving up alcohol, I battled. For quite a few years, my drinking was excessive, and to be honest I could have been on the verge of falling into the deep-end concerning my intake. And if it looks like a problem from the outside, then I am sure it had made me a mess on the inside. Yet giving up alcohol allowed me to keep a clear head for a 40-day period, analyse myself and alter the future that alcohol will have in my life from this day forward.

Change is difficult, and changing requires battling, but change is damn rewarding. My body, my mind and my health have changed. In doing so, I have become a happier person. Change has uncovered a new person and therefore new possibilities in my life. On this very day exactly one year ago, I was battling a birthday hangover just like the prior year's that left me nearly comatose for the day. But, it only took me forty days to understand that in order to take two steps forward in health and fitness, one must take a step back in time, to the City Caveman way of life.

Today, I am fit, I am healthy and I am happier than I have ever been before. I am 35 years old, and I am going for a run in gorgeous Sydney to celebrate my new health, my new beginning and my new life.

Care to join me?

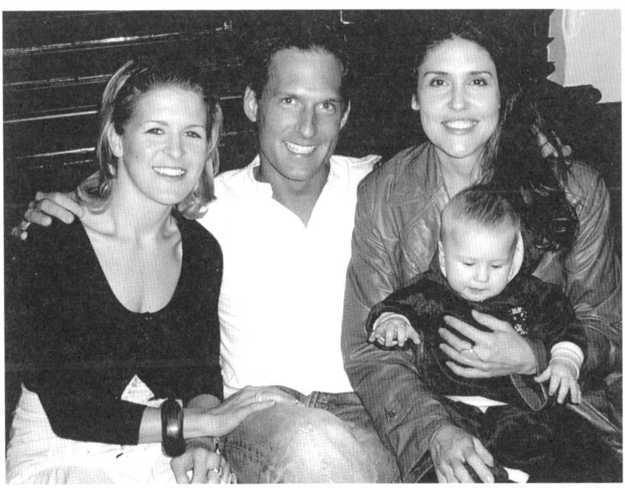

Sonja, me, Annie and Hunter at my 35th birthday party.

Michael Jarosky's transformation continues as he now works in Sydney as a Personal Trainer, guiding others on their *40 Days as a City Caveman* journey. Mike can be found on the Bondi to Coogee run most days and can be contacted on his website:
www.citycavemanfitness.com

Annie Clark and her son Hunter are happy and healthy in Sydney's sunny suburbs. Annie's contact details and purchase information for her fitness DVD 'Getting the Body You Want' can be found on her website:
www.annieclark.com.au

Your Notes